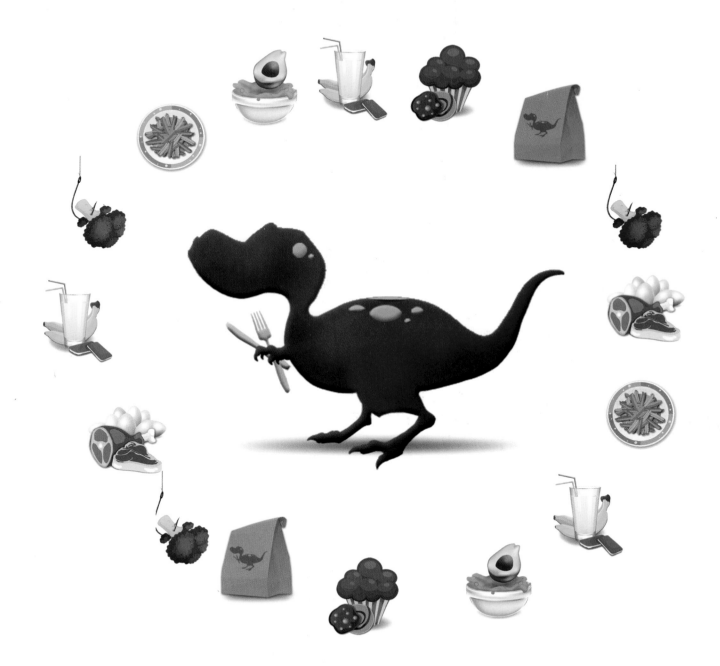

First Published in 2012 by Victory Belt Publishing Inc.

ISBN 13: 978-1-936608-87-4

Photos by Stacy Toth

Eat Like A Dinosaur

By The Paleo Parents

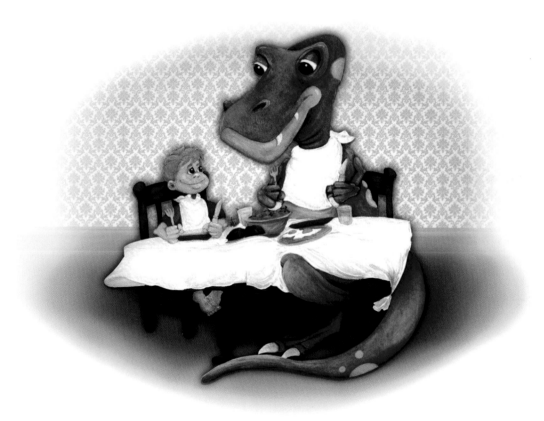

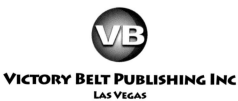

Victory Belt Publishing Inc

Las Vegas

FOR THE ASTRONAUT, THE PIRATE, AND THE NINJA
WITH LOVE

You inspire us to do better, try harder, and be the best we can be. It's your love, happiness, and health that fueled this fire. Thank you for being our "boycheks," and for teaching us how to do handstands again, climb trees, and find toads under rocks.

- Your parents

TABLE OF CONTENTS

THANKS

We heard that writing a book is hard, that your vision gets washed away by those you work with, and that it's even harder to get published. We heard that it takes years or decades for an idea to become a project, for the project to become a book, and for that book to get into a person's hands. We've been lucky enough not to know about any of that. Writing this book has been a whirlwind, and it turned out better than we could have hoped for in mere months.

We have a lot of people to thank for that. It's because of friends, family, and fellow bloggers that our idea grew into a book. Their support and willingness to chat about ideas and taste-test recipes in their homes astounded us. They even sent us to Victory Belt Publishing, which became our biggest supporter in turning this humble, little vision into a "real" book worthy of your bookshelf.

This community, the gluten-free and paleo community, is like nothing else. It's filled with supportive, helpful, open, and giving individuals. We personally know quite a few, all of whom we could never thank enough here, and they are what you would like to imagine them to be. They want to help heal the world, just like us. We will forever be grateful for their willingness to give of themselves and be our silent partners on this endeavor.

A special thanks must go out to one of our first heroes on this journey, Elana Amsterdam, who, despite her own responsibilities at home and on her blog, graciously agreed to write a fantastic foreword that truly moved us. Another thank you must also go to Bill Staley of Primal-Palate.com who brought his big boy camera to our house, some four hours away, to take the family photo featured inside and on the back cover of this book.

Despite all the new friends we've made during this project, it's our old friends and family who we counted on for daily encouragement. Their praise and unyielding support drove us to start a blog. To our friends and family who didn't complain as we ignored them for months, who played with our boys while we spent all day elbows deep in recipe development, you are nothing short of awesome and we are forever grateful. We offer an open invitation to our paleo dinner table.

And to you there, holding this book—you ROCK. Your support and encouragement, your visits to our website, your willingness to try something new and give us a chance, has been our biggest motivator. We only hope the recipes, story, and information in this book are a worthy token of our appreciation and provide what you've been waiting for—a book for your children that helps them feel a little less "different."

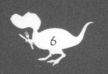

6

Eat Like a Dinosaur

FOREWORD

BY ELANA AMSTERDAM

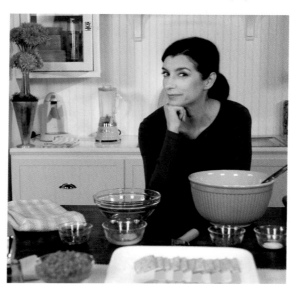

When I was diagnosed with celiac disease in 1998, I went gluten-free in an efficient and matter-of-fact way. Eliminating all of the offending foods, I didn't even try to replace gluten-filled bread with alternative baked goods. I ate very simply and thought nothing of it.

A couple of years later, when my oldest son received the same diagnosis as a toddler, it was an entirely different story. I was upset and in shock—I wanted my little boy to have all of the treats that I had enjoyed growing up. The last thing I wanted was for him to be deprived.

With this in mind, I made it my mission to turn all of my favorite childhood foods into healthy gluten-free classics.

When my son was in elementary school, I used every opportunity I had to make gluten-free treats for his entire class. I soon found myself stopped daily in the school parking lot by parents wanting to get healthy recipes from me—whether their children were gluten-free or not. The requests were rolling in.

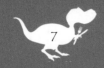

As a result, in 2006, I started my blog (elanaspantry.com) to share my recipes and tips for healthy living with friends and family (and all the parents at school!).

In the following years, I gained great satisfaction helping families make the transition to a healthy lifestyle by continuing my blog and writing two gluten-free, grain-free cookbooks.

Fast forward to early 2011 when the Paleo Parents and I crossed paths. They had begun frequenting my blog—leaving their indelible mark, with numerous helpful comments and friendly ideas for my other readers. Of course I liked them right off the bat.

When Stacy contacted me directly in the summer of 2011 to say that she and Matt not only read and enjoyed my blog, but also wanted me to write the forward for their book, I was thrilled. Why? Synergy.

Our missions are the same—to help people heal themselves from the inside out.

Yet, the Paleo Parents do something different, something very special. They focus on family wellness in a way that is rarely addressed. They are not afraid to talk about the socio-physical-emotional transformation process that true healing entails. This is a formidable task.

I can tell you wholeheartedly, however, that Stacy and Matt are more than up to the challenge. They have written a book that provides not only nourishing grain-free recipes, but also a map for parents wanting to take charge of family healing.

Stacy and Matt set out on an amazing journey in early 2010. Just about one year later, after their family gave up junk food for wholesome fare, moved their fannies off the couch, and lost a collective 200 pounds, they were on the road to vibrant healthy living.

Not only that, Stacy and Matt also healed a myriad of chronic health problems that had been plaguing their children for years, including:

- ADHD
- Childhood Obesity
- Asthma
- Eczema
- Allergies

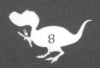

8

In just one year, this couple had become their own health advocates with fantastic results.

In *Eat Like a Dinosaur*, Stacy and Matt share their journey and strategies with you. They simplify complex ideas with statements such as:

Food is nourishment, fuel for our bodies. Think about how your car runs when you put bad gasoline in it.

Ideas such as this make the book a useful manual for life, not just a cookbook full of great recipes.

And yet, great recipes there are. My own children beg for the 50/50 Bacon Burgers, and other healthy, high protein meals that keep their motors running smoothly.

Best of all, you can share (and eat) the recipes in this cookbook with your family too.

Ultimately, this book is a huge contribution to families and children that are in transition with their health and wellness.

Whether you're a beginner just exploring paleo and the grain-free lifestyle or someone like me (I've been strictly grain-free for over ten years), this book deals with everything from how to speak to your children about food and evolving dietary habits to social strategies for dealing with family members and relatives not as accustomed to healthy living and eating.

Stacy and Matt invite you into their home to share a glimpse of the healing system they have created for themselves and their children Cole, Finian, and Wesley.

This darling family is walking, talking proof of how to live better, healthier lives—a good thing in this world of multinational corporations that inundate us with billions of dollars in advertising to promote the processed franken-foods that do not nourish or heal, but actually cause harm.

Many thanks to the Paleo Parents for sharing their touching, healing journey, as well as strategies for not just surviving, but thriving.

KEY

 Throughout this book you will find many recipes where little hands have been placed over certain numbers in the instructions. These are steps that you and your kids can do together. We try to allow our children to do as much as they can in the kitchen, which often means doing steps that some other parents might feel uncomfortable doing. Finian, at three years old, often stirs simmering pots while we let Cole, six years old, chop soft vegetables with a blunted knife. Plus, who doesn't love pushing the 'on' switch on a locked-down food processor? Please use your own judgment about what your child can handle and always use close supervision, especially around hot and sharp things!

With each recipe we've included a notes section for your own use. Here is an example of how you might use it:

Notes:
We really loved this one! Simon was licking his plate!

Notes:
This was a little too spicy. We will take out the ginger the next time we make it.

Notes:
Wanted to make this, but had no palm shortening. Used butter instead and it worked just great!

We've called out the top eight allergens in our recipes as well. If the symbol is highlighted, it means it contains that particular ingredient. If it is gray, it does not contain that ingredient. Here are the symbols:

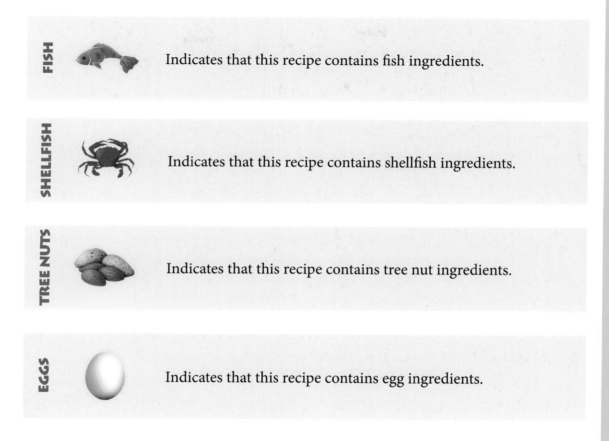

FISH — Indicates that this recipe contains fish ingredients.

SHELLFISH — Indicates that this recipe contains shellfish ingredients.

TREE NUTS — Indicates that this recipe contains tree nut ingredients.

EGGS — Indicates that this recipe contains egg ingredients.

These four allergens are not used in any of the recipes in this book, but their icons have been included on the side of each recipe for reassurance.

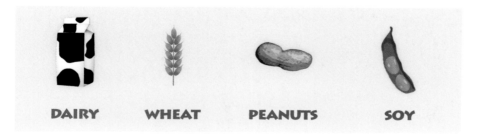

DAIRY   **WHEAT**   **PEANUTS**   **SOY**

Key

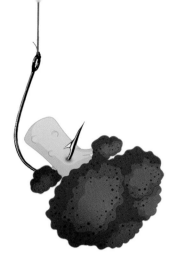

CHAPTER 1
THE BORING CHAPTER FOR PARENTS

Introduction

If you're anything like us, you're already convinced that you should be eating real food instead of the processed food so available these days. You really believe in the health-enhancing benefits of shopping the outside walls of the grocery store. You're on the path to going gluten-free, casein-free, or maybe all allergen-free. Perhaps you've found the Weston A. Price Foundation, or, like us, approach food with an evolutionary premise and eat paleo or primal. So, you've cleaned out your pantry, you've stopped going out to eat so often, and you've started making real food at home.

You've probably started to see and feel significant health gains: lost weight, improved mood, better blood pressure, regulated cholesterol, and general better health. There's only one teensy problem: you have to convince your kids to forget about all their favorite foods and the conventional wisdom they've heard their whole life, in order to join you on this new path.

You're an adult with a strong will and an understanding of the biological impact nutrition can have on your aging body, but a child's interests lie in his or her taste buds. Kids are, after all, much pickier; they're honest to a fault. Food falls into two categories on first glance: it's either edible or disgusting. When they've been enjoying the flavors of pizza and ice cream, suddenly replacing them with spinach and fruit for dessert will probably cause some temper tantrums—even from the teenagers! At the same time, you know that it's best for them to start eating this way.

Believe me, we understand. We have three young kids of our own and have had to change their diet, too. It was a gradual process, but now we have children who can tell us what they should and shouldn't eat, children who know why we eat what we do and who think for themselves about food choices being worth the "cost." It was a molding process, but it's truly been the greatest single thing we've ever done for them and their futures.

We decided to write this book for neither a culinary savant nor a mega-athlete. It's a book for ordinary families who want to start cooking and eating together with their children in a healthful way. After reading this book with your children we hope you'll see that change is possible. It might not be easy, but with a little advice and some enticingly fun-looking recipes, we hope to see you on the other side of the journey. You will have some happy, healthy kids that will love to eat nutrient-dense foods and feel "normal" with our healthier incarnations of old favorites.

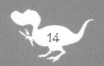

Eat Like a Dinosaur

About Us

Who are we to give advice? We're an average suburban family. We don't have a secret trust fund nor do we have, as you might be hoping to find in this book, a magic spell to make a complete upheaval of long-held beliefs completely painless. We became the Paleo Parents over time. It is still an evolving process that we continue to adapt to in our everyday "normal" life. What we do know is how to take a family from eating poor-quality food of poor nutritional value to eating real, whole foods every meal of the day. It's what we did, and we ended up benefitting tremendously from it.

Because our journey became something that we were excited about and had a passion for, it grew into something we wanted to share. So one evening, on a whim, my wife, Stacy, decided to start a blog. PaleoParents.com was birthed on our humble laptop (missing twelve keys from the toddlers that have enjoyed popping them on and off since we originally brought it home years ago) in our living room. Honestly, we expected only eight friends and some family members to be interested in reading about the wacky thing we were doing that had so drastically changed our lives. We started blogging about our family and how our lives had changed. In hindsight, we realize ours is an interesting story and a powerful testimonial for the positive impact of dietary change.

Based in Fairfax County of Northern Virginia, in the foothills of Capitol Hill, we are a one-income household with two parents and three kids. Our three boys are less than five years apart, so we're the people you see out in public trying to chase after two boys running in opposite directions, shrieking in delight because they know they've got us outnumbered.

Where we are a bit unique is we've upended the traditional gender roles—mom is the one who works and dad is the one who is at home with the children. After the birth of our second son, it wasn't financially reasonable to pay someone to care for the children when my income was bringing in barely more than we'd be paying out. So, I "retired" to take care of our children the way we really wanted. Soon, by necessity, I went from not knowing how to boil water to making every single home-cooked meal the family consumes inside of three years.

As if this choice wasn't odd enough for our circle of friends, somehow we've gone from being the "weird" role-reversed family to the "health nut" family. Acquaintances know we've made huge changes in our lives, but they don't know what, why, or how. Since they seem to always be shocked at our choices for protein, unprocessed fats, and leafy greens (yes, our boys now love spinach), it's nice to have a website to tell people where they can learn more. And now, we're thrilled to be able to do that for you with this book.

The way that we decided to approach diet is called *paleo*. Stacy discovered it after our youngest son was born and, with the help of *The Paleo Diet* by Loren Cordain and *The Paleo Solution* by Robb Wolf, soon converted me as well. Simply put, the paleo diet advocates eliminating all grains, legumes, dairy products, and refined sugar. The idea is that human beings are adapted best to a diet free of these gut irritants. That said, this is not strictly a book about that particular form of eating.

One of the real turning points in our conversion was the discovery of Elana's Pantry, a gluten-free recipe blog run by Elana Amsterdam. She highlighted using almond flour and unrefined sugars to make items we had really been missing, like brownies and cakes. High in protein, low on the glycemic index, and delicious! Once we realized favorite foods didn't have to go away, that they just needed to change a little bit, getting on board became much easier. It is our hope that after reading this book, we can do for you what Elana did for us.

After losing over 200 pounds together in less than fifteen months, as well as transforming our health and that of our children, we don't mind being the family whose children routinely refuse cookies or cake and say "Ew" out loud to cereal and fast-food commercials on TV. It wasn't always this way, of course, and everything we do these days is thanks to our discovery of the paleo way of eating and adapting our modern life to a healthier way of living. Not only has it improved our lives, but the changes in our children have been spectacular as well.

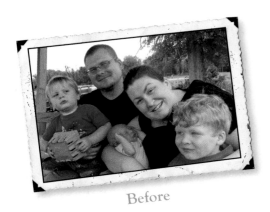

Before

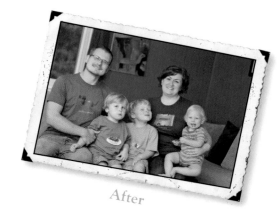

After

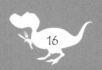

Our Kids

We didn't know it back when we began this journey, but kids can be tremendously helped by diet change. Our kids were not well and we didn't even realize it! Even our (old) pediatrician believed that our boys' ailments were "normal." These days, the norm is acceptance of health ailments rather than finding the root cause of issues through "nutritional therapy." Oh wow, we're such hippies! We use the phrase "nutritional therapy" with you because we assume you won't judge us. We know it's a silly term. We used to mock it, but it's incredibly valid.

Food is nourishment, fuel for our bodies. Think about how your car runs when you put bad gasoline in it. Our poor kids were operating on refined carbohydrates, hydrolyzed wheat proteins, high-fructose corn syrup, and soy additives in almost every meal. And we were eating "healthy" according to the United States government guidelines. No wonder our kids weren't feeling their best! Fortunately, nutritional therapy, or resolving health ailments by eating foods your body wants, brought us to where we are today and gave us three happy, healthy kids.

Cole

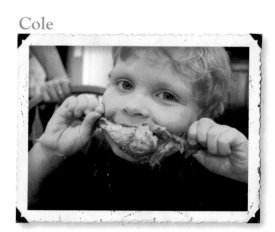

When Cole was an infant, he was the chubbiest baby you have ever seen. A friend once made a joke about not knowing his eye color because his eyelids were so chubby you could hardly see his irises! An entirely breastfed baby, he spent most of his baby and toddlerhood at the 90th percentile for weight and the 25th percentile for length. This was on his mothers grain- and sugar-filled milk. We left our doctors' visits filled with pride about our strong and healthy boy (90% is only 10% away from the goal, right?). Little did we realize how quickly a chubby baby could turn into an overweight preschooler. At three years old his height and weight were unable to be plotted on the doctor's BMI chart, and we struggled with worry and fear that he might have a future defined by weight and health struggles similar to his mother's.

At the same time, Cole was experiencing serious self-control issues. Particularly, and most worrisome, he was hurting his peers with very rough play. In fact, his play-based cooperative preschool came very close to expelling him unless we were able to help him realize that his mind needed to connect with his body. It wasn't that he was mean; everyone knew he was a sweet, well-meaning boy. He just was not able to make his body do what his mind desired because excitement or anger would take over before his mind could regulate his behavior.

When we removed processed foods from his diet (including chemical additives, grains, refined sugar, legumes, and dairy), we immediately saw an improvement in his self-control and ability to listen to authority figures. He went from being a serious safety concern to being called "the best-behaved student in school" almost overnight. It was fantastic to go from getting calls home about "incidents" at school to getting calls home about how wonderful he was. At his first parent-teacher conference in kindergarten, his teacher started describing a student we had always hoped for but never expected to have. What a pleasant surprise!

Over the next year his weight remained steady while his height began to grow, and he moved back onto the BMI chart and into a "normal" range. Additionally, his exercise and cold-induced asthma, which required a daily inhaler, had completely disappeared. Incidents of bed wetting, as often as five times a week, immediately stopped. And a weird rash the doctor's couldn't resolve for several months vanished within weeks.

Cole is our inspiration for this book—we love all our boys with all of our hearts, but seeing the changes in him has inspired us to make the time and effort to share our lessons with the world. There is nothing more astounding than seeing your child struggling with every fiber of his being to behave and succeed in the world, only for the problems to be resolved with some simple nutritional changes. Now the most fervent health evangelist you'll ever meet, Cole loves to teach anyone who will listen about healthy eating. We're constantly hearing him inform his younger brothers, "You can't eat that, it has wheat and dairy!"

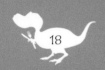

18

Finian

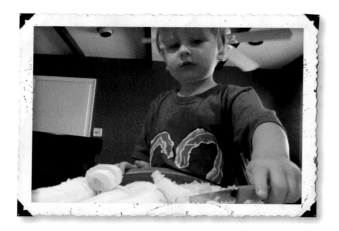

Finian is our most energetic and spirited child. A typical middle child, he strives for our attention in the most simultaneously enthusiastic and exhausting of ways. His joy is contagious and his laughter intoxicating, but, by golly, don't make him frustrated, sad, or angry or you will feel his wrath! Although Finian was only two years old when we removed processed foods from his diet, we've been able to track his remarkable progress by how those "highs" and "lows" have become more normalized.

Finn has always been extremely active, flitting from place to place, seemingly unable to stay on task for very long. You aren't supposed to diagnose attention-deficit disorders until elementary years, but our doctor had already mentioned the possibility by his two-year checkup. Attention deficit runs in my family and has been a serious detriment to at least three boys in my generation. We hoped desperately that Finn would be spared such a fate.

What's amazing about Finian adapting to healthy eating is that his ability to give attention, listen to instructions, and focus his energy in a positive way has improved while his charismatic energy and excitement remains unchanged. The fear we had of our boys becoming medicated zombies is no longer a concern, as Fini is now able to attend our play-based preschool, as well as a "normal" county summer camp program, without any problems. He'll still make up superhero games that involve leaping off tall surfaces and talk so loudly when he's excited that you think your eardrums might burst, but when it's time to sit and read books, he sits there and pays close attention.

And last but not least, Finn seemed to be quickly headed down Cole's medical history path. He was definitely following the top of the weight chart, matching his brother's stats. His issues were compounded by terrible skin sensitivities, eczema all over his body, and fever-inducing pet allergies. As expected, his three-year checkup showed that not only was his weight plotting back on a "normal" range, but his eczema, pet allergies, and overall skin sensitivities had resolved themselves with our diet change as well. He remains sensitive to nightshades (tomatoes, white potatoes, peppers, and eggplants), so we're more careful with his diet than the other two boys, and we use a gentle wash and coconut oil on his skin when he indulges in a ketchup bath.

Wesley

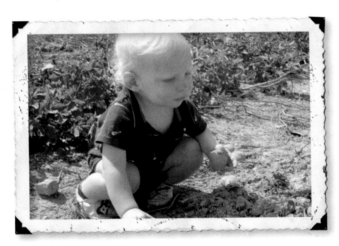

Wesley's birth coincided with Stacy switching her diet. He has had the great fortune of never eating grains or dairy, since Stacy's breast milk never had it, and neither has he had any in his solid foods. For Wes, all we can do is compare him to our experience with the other boys, since we cannot note changes. Wes has, by a noticeable degree, been our most trouble-free, happy baby. He's an easy-going guy, yes. But you're bound to be happier in general when you sleep well, don't have gas, and your skin isn't bothering you.

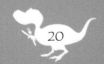

Because Stacy's breast milk has always been gluten-free and casein-free for him, he's never had the serious gas issues that plagued the other two boys when they were infants. Cole had terrible colic, fussiness, and gas for the first few months of life, until Stacy realized it was her consumption of cow's milk that created the issue. I became the baby gas whisperer, always bouncing and rubbing upset tummies the older boys experienced. Wes, however, spends most of his days smiling and laughing and chasing his brothers instead of crying. He's never had gas pain of any kind, in fact.

Wes has barely ever been sick, with only one fever ever (in over 18 months) and no hospitalizations. His oldest brother, Cole, was feverish at least once a month, even hospitalized twice. And Wes has never had the skin sensitivity issues that plague his brother Finian. In fact, Wes hasn't even had so much as a diaper rash. Teething even seems more tolerable. He happily sleeps through the night, and has since an early age (except for quick feedings when he was under a year old). In terms of weight, Wesley has steadily maintained slightly above the 25th percentile and seemingly will never plot outside the chart like his brothers, despite an extraordinary appetite.

Wes will literally eat for hours straight without stopping. Dinner guests gasp as he downs two or three adult-size hamburger patties alongside fruit and veggies for dinner. After eating, he will play as hard as any baby you've ever seen, crawling, and now toddling from one end of the house to the other, causing trouble as he goes. He's alert, happy, and full of his own whippersnapper ninja-like personality, balled up in the mask of an adorable little baby.

How to Get Kids to Love Broccoli

So you're convinced and ready to convert but are confused as to where to start? We've got some tricks up our sleeves and we don't mind sharing. But before we do, it's worth mentioning that kids are highly sensitive to the information you give them. Changing something as fundamental as the food they're used to consuming must be done carefully. Here are our recommendations on how to transition.

Tony Danza Is Not the Boss, You Are!

As the parent, you have tremendous control over what your child eats. When he or she is with you, nothing can go into their mouth without you having some part of approving it. This is of course true of the very young; Wesley, until recently, couldn't

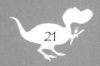

reach any food, let alone know how to access it once he got there. But even when they are older, you are still in charge of what food is kept in your house. This makes the easiest step in converting your children obvious: remove the unhealthy foods from your house and they will no longer be an option.

Now, obviously, we don't all have full control. Some households don't have both parents on board, and some parents share custody in different households, often leading to one parent undermining the efforts of the other. Ideally, the "normal diet" parent would respect the ideas of his or her other half as it relates to food. After all, most of the real-food principles are hard to argue against. What rational parent would disagree with the idea that less chemical-based food and more fresh foods benefit health? You will often be able to make compromises with your partner parent so that the kids are fed healthy foods more often than not. But for the problem areas, you will likely have to accept that there will be some occasions where you will not have control over your kids' diet and they will eat less healthy.

Our boys love to visit grandparents, and there they're spoiled with foods we request not to know about. We encourage the host to help our children make good choices, we remind them of what is and isn't appropriate, and we always pack our child's favorite snacks in their bag. Our hard-and-fast request is absolutely no gluten. We beg and plead. We bribe. The most effective tool, though, has been fear mongering: tell the host the truth, "Just remember, he's not used to having sugar and gluten. If you give him those things, he will most likely be bouncing off the walls and then crashing with a tummy ache—which doesn't make your time together very fun." That has seemed to really make the difference in hosts attempting to comply. Cole comes home and tells me they had eggs and bacon for breakfast (instead of pancakes) but did have ice cream— "without cookies in it!" To us, that is success.

After your kids become used to eating this way and understand why the change is important, they will start telling people what they can and can't eat on their own. One of our favorite stories we've been told is of a divorced couple that had different diet ideas. Once the mother had successfully converted her children's diet, the kids started telling their dad that they would NOT be eating pizza with him. After a while, he switched over as well!

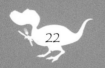
22

Transition Quickly; Be Prepared to Make Concessions

We feel that you will have more success with your children if the decision to change their diet is a sudden change instead of a drawn-out process in which they lose their favorite foods. Kids like routine and rules, and they just need you to give them the rules (and the rationale, depending on age) and then stick with them. Really, stick with them. You cannot be willy-nilly on things as a parent because children sense your weakness!

You'll get push-back the first time they are told Friday pizza night is now off the table (preface it with "in this house" if you need to). But if you pull out this book or other material to help them learn why pizza hurts their bodies and you really stick with it, they'll accept it eventually. Especially if Friday night becomes International Food Night or Breakfast for Dinner Night instead! If right away you establish their new guidelines, they will know what to expect and be more ready to accept the individual choices this entails.

Consider that you yourself like to have treats: that anniversary dinner, the marshmallow while camping, the donut while you visit your hometown. The key to successful parenting is to remember that your child is his or her own person. Kids are born into this world with their own personality, and as parents we hope they'll continue to have it until after we're gone. If your child is begging you for a treat, figure out a way to make it happen. Just make sure it stays occasional and call it a "special treat" so that everyone recognizes it's not good food.

None of this is to say that you shouldn't feel free to make their new diet as familiar or comforting to them as possible. When we first transitioned our kids we still made occasional sandwiches on gluten-free bread and let them eat quinoa pasta when they were lamenting their loss. This helped them feel like the world wasn't ending, and it gave us an opportunity to talk about what was different about those foods from what we usually ate. Eventually, those things stopped being asked for and they got used to their new way of eating. It was a proud moment when we saw our kids remove their gluten-free bread and eat the veggies and meat from the middle of their sandwich!

Do NOT Force Your Child to Eat Anything

We recommend encouraging children to eat a little bit of everything on their plate. Of course they're going to gobble up applesauce before they touch the kale. However, it's quite logical to explain that before they have more applesauce, they try one bite of protein and vegetables. Even the three year old is able to grasp the concept of balancing out a meal when we encourage him to just try one bite of his vegetables. If he chooses not to, that's OK, we will not force him. It just means he's not starving, and he doesn't have to have more applesauce in order to fill himself up.

Some foods just won't appeal to your children. Remember: their taste buds are different from yours and taste everything more strongly than yours do. Very young children even have an enzyme difference (salivary amylase) in how their saliva breaks down food, causing dietary starches (like broccoli) to not break down into sugar in their mouth (get sweeter as you chew it), which is what happens in adults.

There is a reason they don't like certain foods. What they dislike will surprise you just as much as what they will like! One of our kids loves greens like spinach and kale and yet will not eat oranges. Another loves avocado more than anything else but won't touch the stems of any green vegetables. Let them dislike foods they've tried. You will always have more success if mealtime is not a battle of wills but a fun experimenting time.

Lastly, the best trick of all: let them dip! This book has quite a few dip and sauce recipes, and that's because dipping is a favorite activity of kids—heck, even adults love to dip! Give your children the choice of which dip they'd like to try with their carrots and you'll likely be surprised at the quantity of carrots that get consumed as they use them as spoons. Just make sure to be up-front as to the quantity of dip or sauce they'll get on a plate, otherwise they'll lick it off the carrot instead of eating it with the vegetable. We like to say, "OK, one spoonful of sauce for what you have on your plate." Then they can logically ration it out and ask for more veggies and sauce together. If your kids love dip, try Mock-A-Mole (p. 139) and our Black Olive Tapenade (p. 141). Because they're made from vegetables with natural, healthy fats, eating a bowlful is only brain food for your kids!

Kids Aren't Going to Let Themselves Starve!

One of the worries we've heard a lot is, "But my kid won't eat any of this stuff! I've got to feed him something!" Granted, what we're about to say is much more apparent

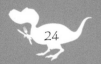

Eat Like a Dinosaur

the younger your kids are, but trust us when we say that no child has ever starved in front of an abundant food supply. As it was recently pointed out to us, there are not picky eaters in third world countries. There may be meals or foods that your child will never eat, but if you continue to put healthy food in front of them, they'll eventually get hungry enough to eat it.

This is not to say that they won't try to convince you otherwise. Kids know how to put on just the right show to get exactly what they want and they've literally been studying how to do it all their lives. What makes their manipulation so convincing is that they actually fully believe what they are telling you, regardless of how unreasonable it actually is.

No matter what they say in a whiny, pleading voice, eating pork chops and asparagus will not harm them, nor will skipping dinner starve them. You are not a bad guardian for asking them to eat healthful, real food. Chicken nuggets and French fries will not cure whatever sickness they are purporting to have. The good news is we've got versions of almost any food they miss (sorry, mac and cheese is going to have to be a box of Annie's Gluten-Free—we got nothin').

One of Stacy's most successful tactics is, "We know eggplant isn't your favorite, but it's what we picked out at the store and Daddy spent a lot of time making this dinner. If you don't even try it and you say it's yucky, how do you think that makes him feel?" Turn that manipulation right back around on them and see where it lands you. But you have to believe it, too. How are you supposed to convince them if right now you are thinking, "That will never happen! There's no way my kid will ever eat kale." If you don't even believe it yourself, it'll never happen for them.

Get Your Child Involved in Food

The more connected your children are to their food, the more willing they will be to eat it and understand why they're eating it. Whenever we can, we take our kids to farms and markets and let them pick out fruits and vegetables. We take them to the store with us, and when in the kitchen, we let them stir the pot. The more involved they are in the preparation of a meal, the more they'll want to eat it. You'll notice that each recipe in this book highlights what kids can do to help. That's because incorporating children into the creative process excites them.

We've cooked things many parents couldn't imagine their child eating. Some of the boys' favorite dishes are unusual foods that are made exciting by the exploration and fun we had finding them. Ox tail, octopus, and mussels are some of their absolute favorites—cooking these unique foods offer an opportunity to teach while cooking with the boys. Then they're so intrigued by what they watched being prepared, they need to taste it.

Getting involved doesn't just mean cooking, though. We are constantly engaging them intellectually about what food is. Our kids know what animal each kind of meat is and they know where different cuts come from. They know why certain foods are good for them and why certain foods make them sick. Every child, no matter the age, is able to learn about nutrition and food. Give them the information at the level they're ready for and let them ask questions from there.

At the end of a long day of playing, nothing is more enjoyable to your child than a tasty, fun meal to eat. As long as you remember that eating is always pleasurable and never a chore, you and your child should quickly learn that eating healthfully is even more pleasing than eating junk.

Tools and Ingredients for Your Kitchen

You may be surprised by some of the ingredients and tools that we use in this book, as some of them are a little unusual. The "supply list" may be a little overwhelming at first and will certainly seem expensive if taken as a whole. I assure you that other than meats, fruits, and vegetables, nothing in the following list needs to be purchased right away. The various tools and ingredients are by no means necessary, but they will be nice to have eventually. Where applicable, we've put alternative ingredients and instructions in our recipes so that you can still make the food without the specializations.

Tools We Find Helpful
Dehydrator

We love to give beef jerky and dried fruit as snacks to our kids. Unfortunately, much of the commercially available products are loaded with chemicals, soy, wheat, and sugar. Quality jerky can be purchased, but it's not cheap—especially when one of your kids can down a whole bag in one sitting.

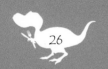

Our solution was to buy a dehydrator. The idea was intimidating at first, but then we realized a dehydrator is just a warm fan with tiers of trays on top and a lid. When you make it yourself, you control the ingredients. In this book there are recipes for several types of jerky, as well as fruit leather roll-ups and dried apples. After several hours, the food is dried out. While it's optimal to switch the trays around for even drying, you can just leave it on overnight and it'll be done in the morning—doesn't get much simpler.

A dehydrator, for a kitchen appliance, is relatively inexpensive. Our mid-grade brand offers a quicker cooking time than the lowest tier, but still it only cost us $40–$50 dollars. We saved that in one month's worth of jerky; we get a lot of use out of it! It's almost a daily occurrence to walk into our house and hear the soft fan of our dehydrator at work.

Food Processor

One of the most versatile tools we have in the kitchen is a food processor. Everything is made so much easier when you don't have to spend all your time mincing every ingredient into tiny pieces. Not only that, but most food processors also have a grater attachment to grate your carrots or zucchini or cabbage. Our kids much prefer grated carrots in their salad to medallions, and of course it makes it easier for baking with veggies!

While by no means is a food processor a requirement, it is very useful and more affordable than you think. While a new one would cost you $30–$60, we always find them at yard sales and thrift stores for under $10. It would be a wise investment to purchase one at that price. You'll make up for it in saved time.

Ice Cream Maker

Ice cream was a religion in our house. We loved to try out new flavors and new brands of ice cream. We're sure many of you would share our pain if you had to walk away from that entirely. At first we tried to fill the void with fruit sorbet or store bought coconut milk ice cream, but they contain quite a bit of sugar. You can solve this dilemma with a simple machine. Modern-day ice cream makers are electric, have bowls you can place in the freezer beforehand (instead of using salted ice), and only take twenty minutes or so to churn.

With an ice cream maker in hand, coconut milk ice cream or real fruit sorbet is just waiting for you! You can buy a good ice cream maker for only $40 or find one at a thrift store for under $10. Best of all, your kids will love to watch as the ice crystals form and the flavored liquid they just mixed up turns into ice cream!

Silicone Muffin Cups

The most common gluten-free baking staples, almond flour and coconut flour, don't rise very well, so you'll likely find yourself making cupcakes and muffins instead of cakes. We found ourselves going through so many paper liners that it seemed prudent to get reusable muffin cups. Silicone sticks to the food less than paper, plus it's nonreactive, so there is even less chemical transfer! A dozen silicone cups can be purchased for about $5 at your local Home Goods or Marshalls.

Electric Stand Mixer

The biggest time saver in our kitchen is certainly our electric stand mixer. They are not cheap (a KitchenAid classic mixer starts at $180, a lesser brand is under $100), but you will find yourself using it all the time. And electric stand mixers are safer and easier for the kids to use than an electric beater. Any batter we make goes into the mixer. Any time we need to whip something, it goes in the mixer. Plus, with the KitchenAid brand you can purchase attachments to do a variety of other functions, like grind meat. For all of our recipes you could use an electric hand mixer for the same purposes. They're under $20 and kids love using them with your help, too. Point is, if you ever want to beat egg whites, you'll appreciate having something!

Meat Grinder

We bought a meat grinder attachment for our stand mixer thinking it would be a neat experiment. But from the moment we ground bacon for our 50/50 Bacon Burgers (p. 51), it became indispensible. You'll appreciate having one, especially if you'd like to start integrating organ meats. Nutrient-dense and affordable pastured organ meat can be made more palatable by adding it into your ground beef. Plus, making your own sausages or hotdogs can be a great project with the kids—and you get to save money in the long-run. There are hand-cranked versions of meat grinders, but whichever way you go

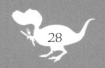

it'll likely run you about $40. Most butchers will grind, slice, or dice any meat you buy, too—so feel free to ask for your livers already ground!

Our Funny Ingredients
Fats and Oils

One of the hardest adaptations for us in the kitchen was replacing oils. Both of us had been raised on canola and vegetable oil. These are highly processed, extracted with chemicals, bleached and oxidized "foods" coming from grains. Unfortunately, these flavorless and easy to work with oils were difficult to replace. But, we found it could be done!

Although we almost always use coconut oil, we use olive and macadamia oil as well. In addition, we frequently use fats: palm shortening, lard, and bacon fat. If you're still not gung-ho about unprocessed fats being healthy, there are tons of resources available online to help you understand how dietary cholesterol is a requisite in your body for brain growth, hormone regulation, and proper absorption of Vitamin D.

Our kids no longer need sun block unless they're out for an entire day in direct sunlight, and our cholesterol blood tests amaze our physicians. But we're not writing this book as experts on any topic other than having fun with your kids in the kitchen. So please look into it yourself and we hope you find that the sources we've chosen are right for your family, too. If not, substitute according to your desires—just choose a solid (fat) or liquid (oil) accordingly.

Coconut oil has all the wonderful gut-healing and healthy fat (repeat after me, saturated fat is not scary) properties of coconut milk, and it is a very flavorful oil for baking or sautéing. It is a solid at room temperature, so when using it keep in mind it will return to that state if given the chance. Coconut oil is available at most stores these days, but look for a brand that has been pressed; it involves less chemical processing than brands that have been solvent extracted. We also love using coconut oil spray, made by Spectrum and available at our local Whole Foods, the same way we used to use Pam for oiling baking sheets. Of course you could always do what your grandmother did and grease it with a towel and some solid coconut oil or lard.

Do not be afraid of lard! We get lard by the tubful from our local farmer's market and use it in everything from pan-frying to giving mashed vegetables a creamy, buttery taste. Real fresh lard is much more delicious than seed oil alternatives. Best of all, it's usually not much more expensive than a similar volume of canola oil, and it stores for a very long time chilled.

For baking in recipes that would normally require butter or shortening, we have replaced seed oil shortening (your Crisco, for example) with palm shortening. Unlike vegetable oil shortenings, there are no trans fatty acids with palm shortening. We buy ours from Tropical Traditions, an online store, but this should be widely available at your local health food store or Whole Foods by the brand Spectrum.

If you are struggling with the idea that fats don't necessarily make you fat and that the right fats can be good for you, we really recommend you read up on the subject from a variety of sources you trust—both from the paleo camp and the standard diet camp—and see where logic puts you. For us, that was how we personally came to the realization that fat is a necessary component for healthy brain development, both in children and adults. There's a reason fish oil is a supplement. From our research, it's our opinion that other foods, like grains and sugar, are the true cause of modern diseases such as heart disease, obesity, and diabetes.

Coconut Milk and Coconut Cream Concentrate

Coconut is one of our favorite foods. We've discussed that it's a healthy fat, but it's also incredibly nutritious and has properties to help heal the gut. Stacy no longer has a gallbladder (a common occurrence for people with gluten intolerance), and the introduction of coconut has helped her digestion immensely.

Coconut milk is the meat of a coconut grated and squeezed to produce a thick milky substance. It has become such a staple in our house that we buy it by the case through Amazon's Subscribe & Save program. It's perfect for replacing milk and cream in your diet, and it works great in certain recipes, such as curries. We have made a faux béchamel sauce out of it with no problem, and have even made a creamy tomato soup. While it does have a coconut flavor, I assure you it's not overpowering. Coconut will fade as the base of your palate with time; no one complains about a milky or buttery flavor, after all.

Please note, in recipes that call for coconut milk, we recommend only full-fat and guar gum–free coconut milk.

A company called Tropical Traditions makes a product called coconut cream concentrate (other brands call it coconut butter). It is the dried and ground coconut meat

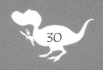

with coconut oil. Reconstituting this will give you control over the thickness of your coconut milk, or you can just add it in directly for a coconut flavor. We suggest you buy these products through Amazon's Subscribe & Save program or through local whole-sale co-ops with whole-food companies for the best deals; they're worth every hefty penny you have to spend and last a long time.

Almond Flour, Coconut Flour, and Other Wheat Replacements

When switching their diet, people often think that they have to entirely eliminate baked goods. This is not true! I can't imagine how our children might react if they could never have a cookie again. While health-friendly baking is a more creative process, it is certainly possible, more healthful, and we believe even more delicious!

The flours we use are blanched almond flour (Honeyville) and coconut flour (Tropical Traditions). And when these flours are too thick for something to rise, we use tapioca flour (Bob's Red Mill). Just as you might expect, these are ground almonds, coconut, and cassava root, respectively. Not only do almond and coconut flours add protein and fat, but they are also much more flavorful than wheat.

Unfortunately, these are a little harder to find, and don't even try to compare the cost to wheat flour (which is subsidized enormously to keep it cheap). Keep in mind, these are "treats," and you'll use much less quantity. While any of these can be acquired easily online, you may need to go to a Whole Foods or a specialty health market to find them in the real world. Alternatively, you can make your own almond or coconut "meal," which is a bit more course but still does the trick, with either a food processor or a powerful blender.

Almond and Sunflower Butter

We use almond butter in quite a few recipes because it's easy to cook with. Honestly, it's our way of cheating when we bake. MaraNatha and Trader Joe's almond butters are our favorites, but any brand will do. Roasted or raw, crunchy or creamy—it's your preference. We suggest raw/creamy for baking and roasted/crunchy for eating. When we use almond butter in a recipe, you can easily make this nut-free by using MaraNatha brand sunflower butter (we suggest adding a bit more oil or fat than called for too). This is a fun experiment for anyone to try, since the chlorogenic acid (chlorophyll) in sunflower seeds reacts with the baking soda when baked, causing the your baked goods to turn green (what fun)!

Arrowroot Powder

Because nut flours don't have the binding proteins that wheat or rice flours do, we use arrowroot as a thickening agent. It works similarly to cornstarch, except it is not a grain; it is made from the tuber of the arrowroot plant, which originated in the tropics. It can be found in most health foods stores and Asian markets, or Bob's Red Mill brand is available online. For the volume you need, it is an affordable product that will last a long time.

Dark Chocolate

Just because you've decided to eat healthier doesn't mean you have to say goodbye to chocolate! Chocolate is made from the fat of the cocoa plant, cocoa butter, and cocoa powder. In fact, good quality chocolates have been shown to offer excellent health benefits because they're high in antioxidants—yippee! Everything else is just additives, so read labels. Our recommendation is to find the darkest (over 70% is best) chocolate you can (our kids even like 90% when we use it in things like our Nut Butter Cups) and try for a brand that's soy- and dairy-free.

You can melt and sweeten Baker's unsweetened chocolate extremely inexpensively, but we like the convenience of Enjoy Life brand mini chips and Dagoba brand; we get them online for the best price. Soy-, wheat- and dairy-free chocolate chips are also available at Whole Foods. Just don't overdo it. Once sugar and starch are no longer a big part of your diet, a tiny amount of chocolate will go a long way for you!

Sweeteners

Palm sugar is an unrefined sweetener with a low glycemic index made from the nectar of the coconut palm, so it even has vitamins and minerals. We use it because it comes granulated and is much more familiar and easier to adapt to traditional recipes. You could, as we often do, grind it into a superfine sugar in a coffee grinder for frostings and meringues. There have been speculations that palm sugar may not be a sustainable food and could affect overall coconut production, so if you're looking for an alterna-

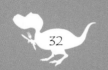

tive, you could use unrefined cane sugar instead. When we bake for ourselves, we prefer maple syrup, honey, ripe bananas, or dates for natural unprocessed sweeteners that offer a depth of flavor not found in standard American sweeteners. Each sweetener we use offers not just unique flavor profiles, but they also include different sucrose and fructose ratios, as well as vitamins and minerals.

Bulk Nuts

If you were to go into our pantry right now, you'd find a giant box on the pantry floor filled with nothing but bags of nuts. We seem to keep every variety on hand; right now we're carrying walnuts, almonds, macadamias, pecans, hazelnuts, Brazil nuts, cashews, and pistachios. Even if you don't cook with them, they make great, quick snacks for your kids.

Just be sure not to overdo your nuts. While walnuts and macadamias have a healthier balance of Omega-6 and Omega-3 fats, all the others are much higher in Omega-6, which can skew some of the progress you've made in going gluten-free or grain-free.

Coconut Aminos, Tamari and Fish Sauce

We love cool, flavorful food. Usually that includes at least one Asian-inspired dish a week. Since the number one ingredient in most soy sauce is wheat, it's absolutely out.

Tamari is soy sauce without wheat, and it's cheap and easy to find at any Asian market. However, it is made with (fermented) soy, and we really try to keep all legumes out of our diet. So we use Coconut Aminos, which is fermented coconut that replicates a similar flavor. It's not cheap, but it should be available at your health food store or Whole Foods.

Fish sauce is made of awesome. Don't be afraid. Well, be afraid of the ones with labels you can't read and hydrolyzed wheat protein as an ingredient. Other than that... get over the fact that you think it smells bad and seems gross. As you will experience with some of the upcoming dishes, it gives the food that "pop" you've been missing. Stacy likes to joke that it's the paleo version of MSG. It's THAT good.

So, parents, you're in the fridge checking your labels and tossing your old, unhealthy foods, when your child asks you what you're doing. When you explain that you're throwing out food, they ask you why you are doing that. Now you're stymied. How can you explain this whole concept to a four year old who has no conception of healthy food, having been marketed sugar cereals, candy, and fast food for all his life? When he has no knowledge of biochemistry or evolutionary biology, how can you explain to him that the food he eats is making him sick?

Well, we wrote this story to help you explain just that. The concept of "eating like a dinosaur" is a simple one to understand and explain to children of any age, and it perfectly encapsulates what you are trying to teach. Children get dinosaurs; they eat meat and they eat vegetables. What they don't eat is bread or candy or beans or anything frozen in a box. We explained to our guys that if we could feed it to a pet Allosaurus or Triceratops, we could put it in our recipes. These days, they use this explanation to anyone who asks about their food: "We only eat what a dinosaur would eat!"

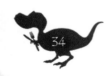

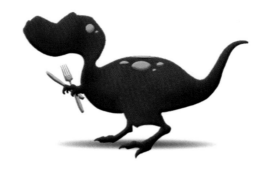

CHAPTER 2

"EAT LIKE A DINOSAUR"

Written by Matthew McCarry & Stacy Toth

Illustrated by Amanda Gates

Told by Cole

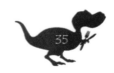

I don't eat the same lunch as most of my friends. And I don't participate in pizza Fridays or breakfast for lunch at school. What I do get is to do something even more special.

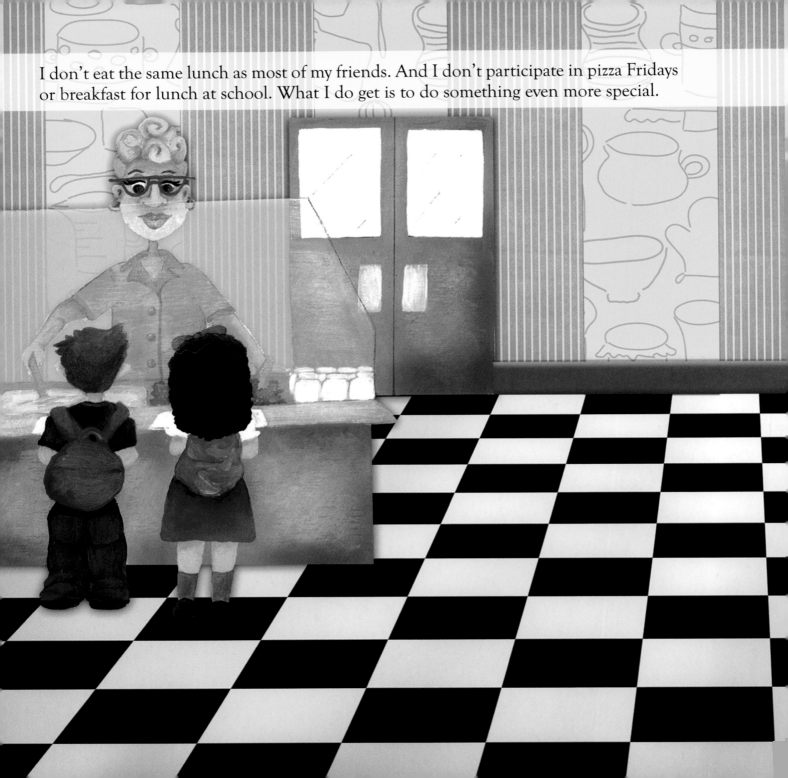

My family and I, we're different because of the way we eat. We eat plants. Dinosaurs like plants. We eat meat. Dinosaurs love meat!

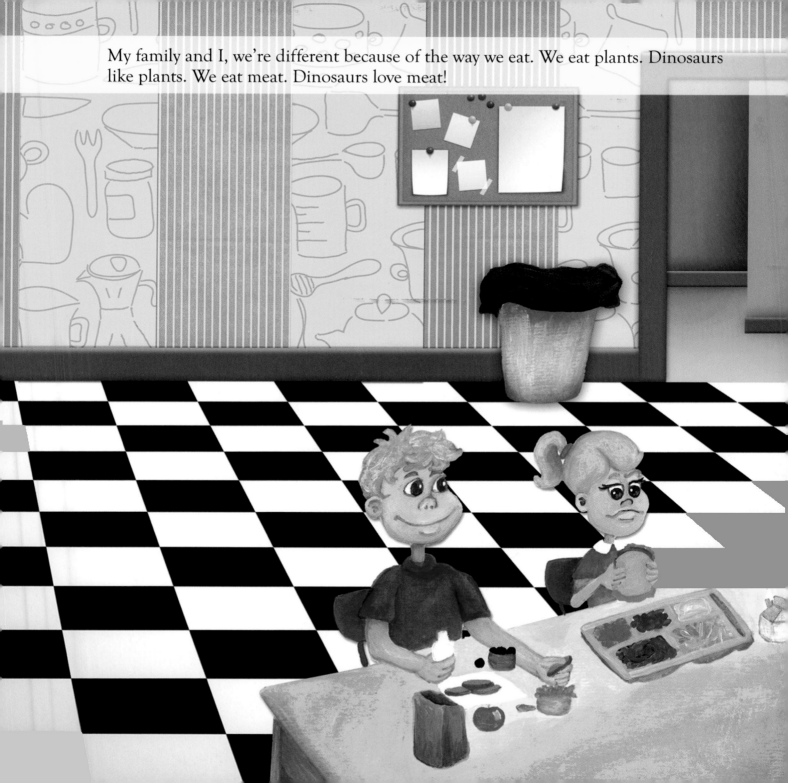

Back in old times, when I was four, my family was a little sick. Some of us were sad a lot of the time. Some of us couldn't control our bodies and got in trouble at school. I even had to take medicine to help my breathing, and my brother had bumps all over his body that never went away! Mostly, though, we were really tired and didn't want to do much except watch TV.

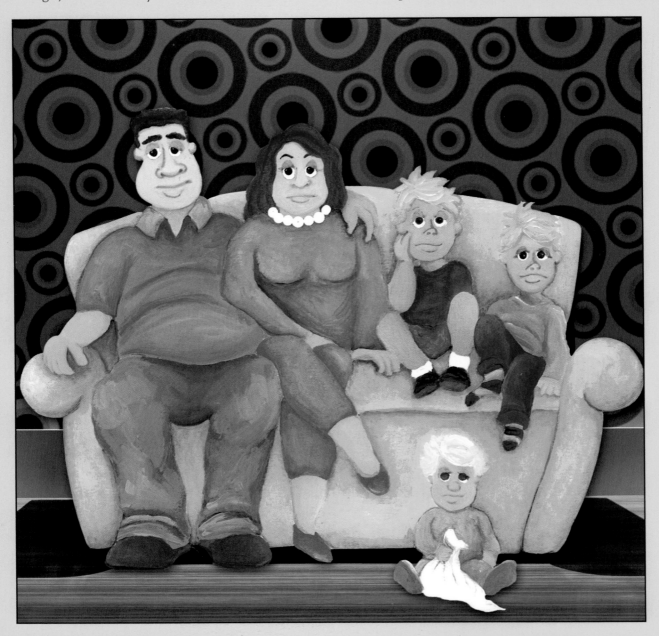

Then my mom got an idea! What if we turned back time and started eating healthy things that we could find in the wild? What if we...ATE LIKE DINOSAURS? You see, dinosaurs didn't make cookies. They didn't eat pasta or bread. They never drank juice boxes or soda. They didn't drink milk or eat cheese. Dinosaurs only ate meat, fruits, and vegetables.

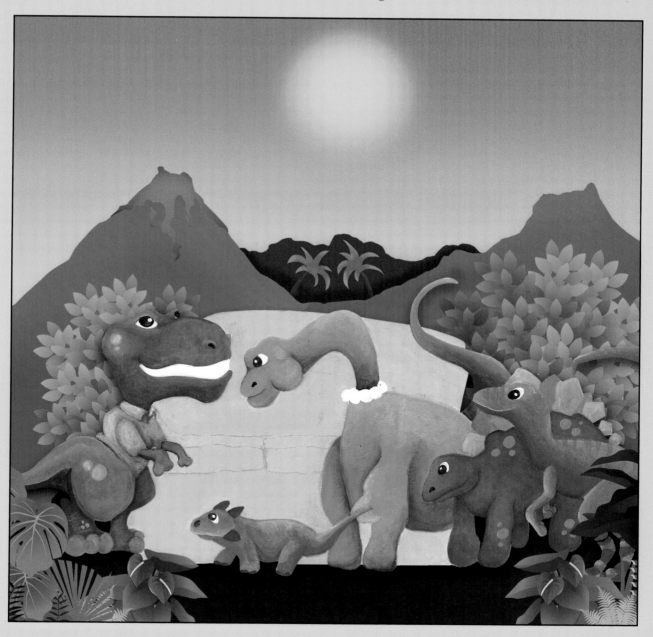

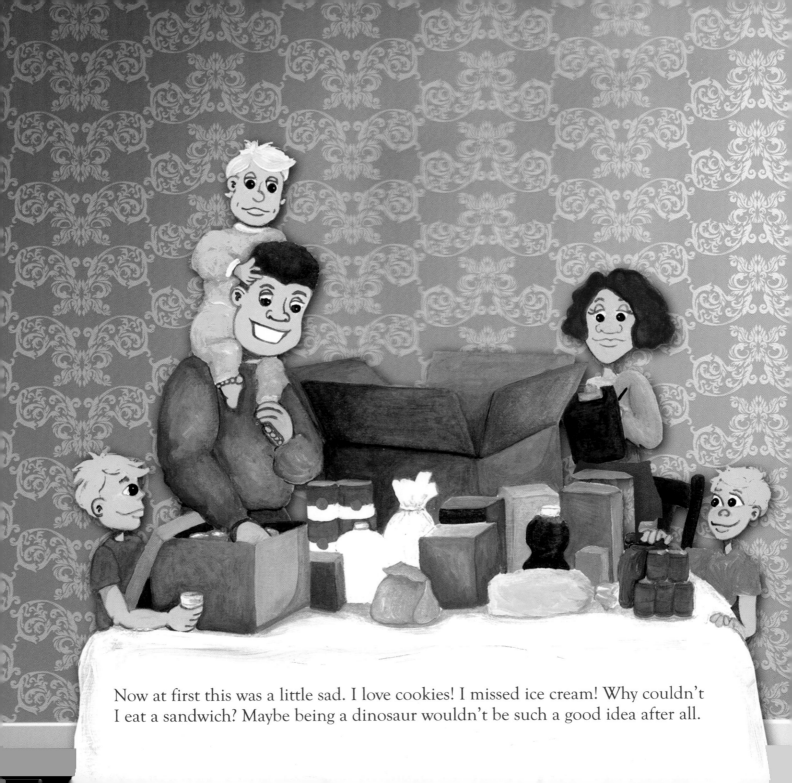

Now at first this was a little sad. I love cookies! I missed ice cream! Why couldn't I eat a sandwich? Maybe being a dinosaur wouldn't be such a good idea after all.

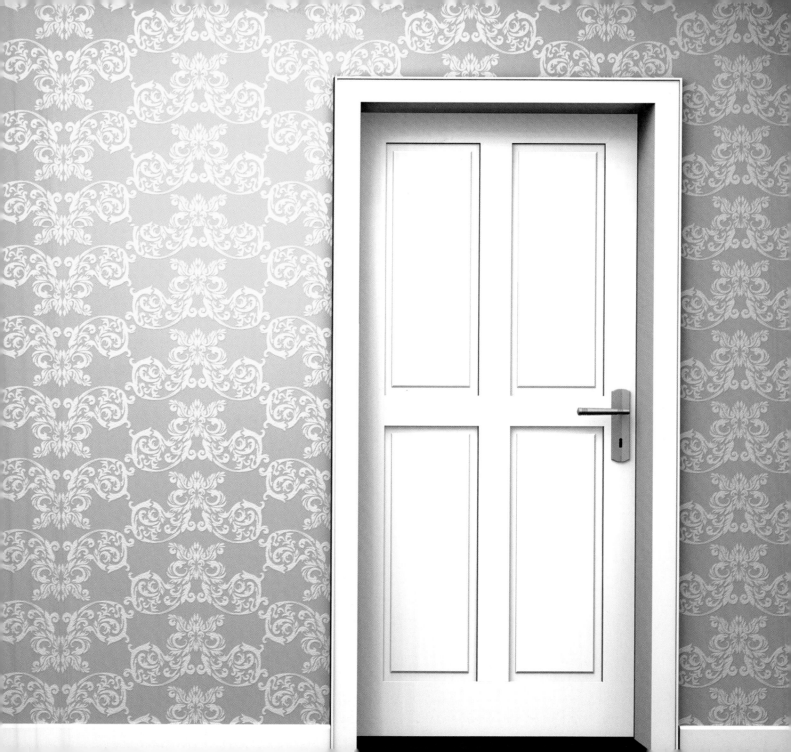

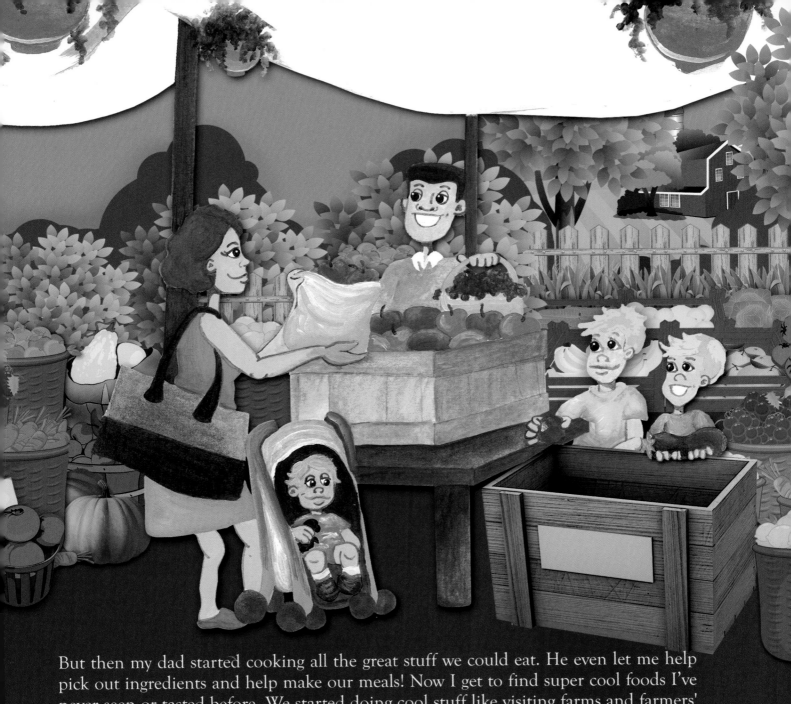

But then my dad started cooking all the great stuff we could eat. He even let me help pick out ingredients and help make our meals! Now I get to find super cool foods I've never seen or tasted before. We started doing cool stuff like visiting farms and farmers' markets, trying out new foods, and trying to think up new ways to make our old foods.

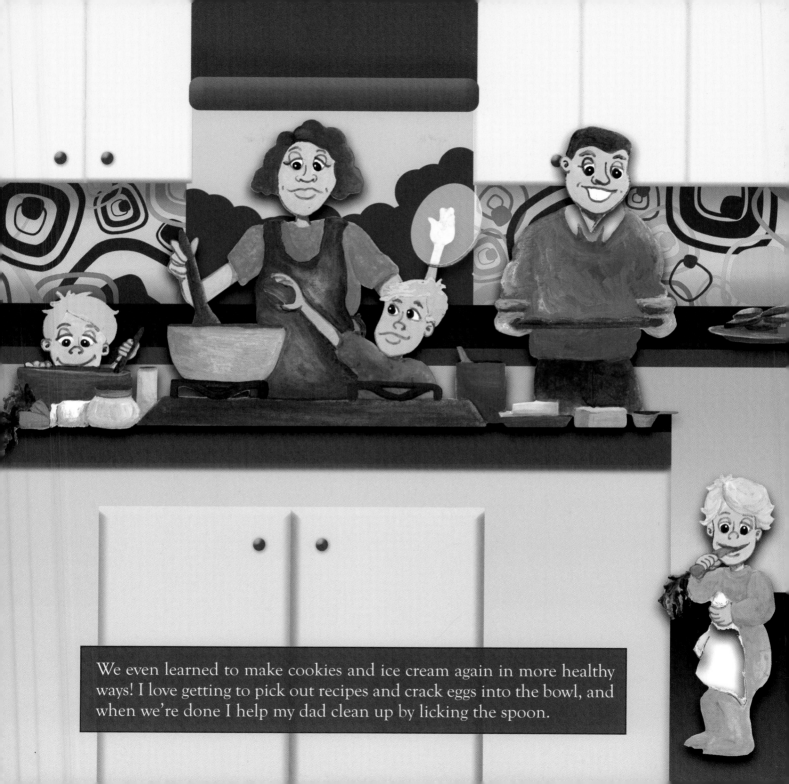

We even learned to make cookies and ice cream again in more healthy ways! I love getting to pick out recipes and crack eggs into the bowl, and when we're done I help my dad clean up by licking the spoon.

Before I could say "Stegosaurus!" my entire family was feeling healthy and strong while also enjoying the new foods we got to eat. I started growing strong like a T-Rex and tall like a Brachiosaur. Hey, maybe this would be fun after all!

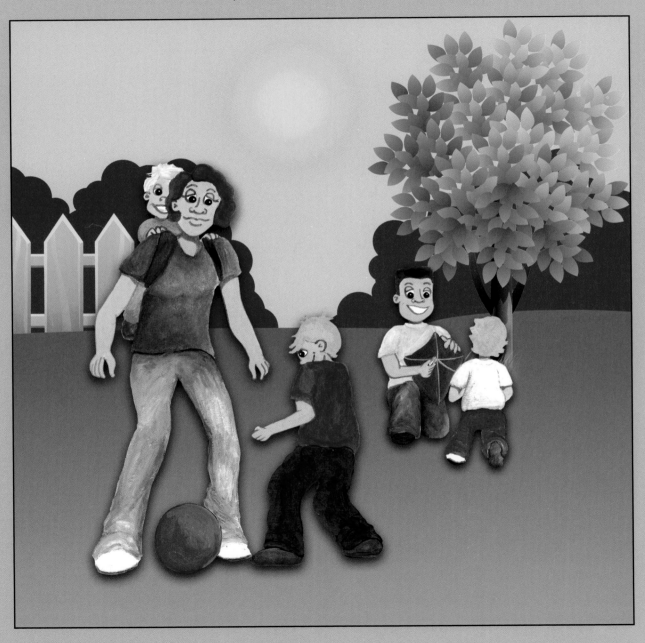

Now we enjoy going out and doing fun stuff instead of feeling sad inside our house. I started getting awards for good behavior in school, got to stop taking my medicine, and my brother's bumps finally went away!

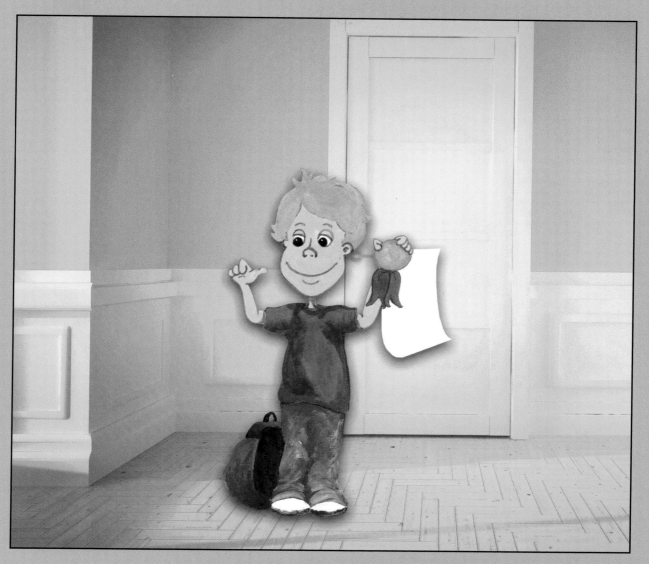

It's not always easy to make the right choices, though. Sometimes I don't realize foods have wheat or dairy hiding in them. If I'm feeling sad or frustrated, I tell my parents and then we make a special treat I can have.

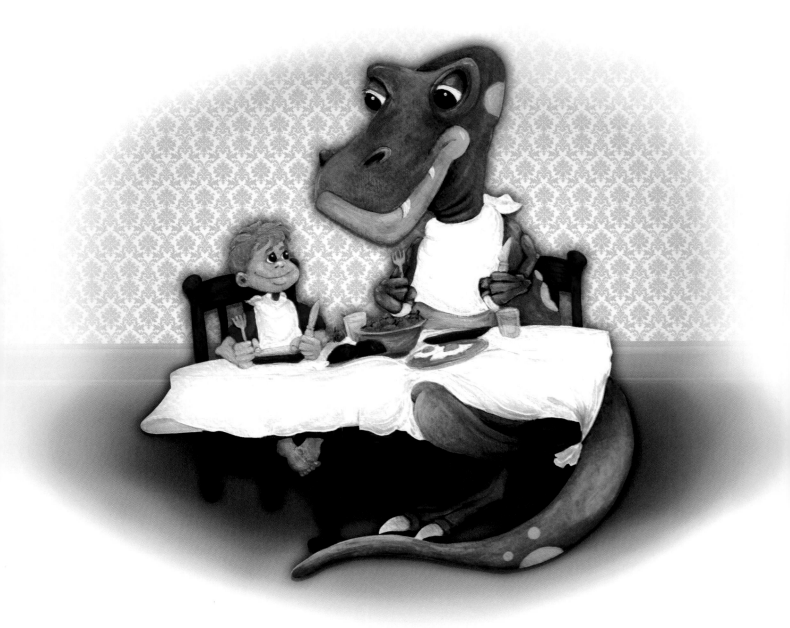

But usually I just ask myself if a dinosaur could eat it.

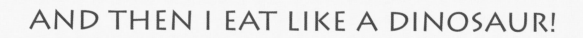

AND THEN I EAT LIKE A DINOSAUR!

We have a little secret for you. You know how sometimes someone will refer to eggs as a "breakfast food" or to steak as a "dinner food"? Well, throw that thought away! When you eat like a dinosaur, all food is anytime food as long as it's healthy!

Do you like omelets? You know, eggs with stuff rolled up inside? We often make that for dinner. Do you like hamburgers? We love them so much we sometimes have them for breakfast! How about fish like salmon or tuna? We love fish for lunch! It doesn't matter when you make something because your belly can't tell time!

Next time you're looking for something to eat, listen to your body and it will tell you what you want to eat. If you want a pork chop with an apple before school, maybe that's something you can have! If you want bacon and eggs for dinner, eat it!

This part of the book is about main dishes, which make up the biggest part of any meal. It could be an egg dish. It could be a meat dish. It could even be a soup. All of the recipes in this section will teach you how to make some delicious and healthy food that dinosaurs would have loved to eat as the big part of their breakfast, lunch, or dinner.

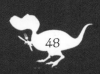

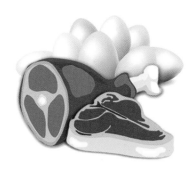

CHAPTER 3
MAIN DISHES

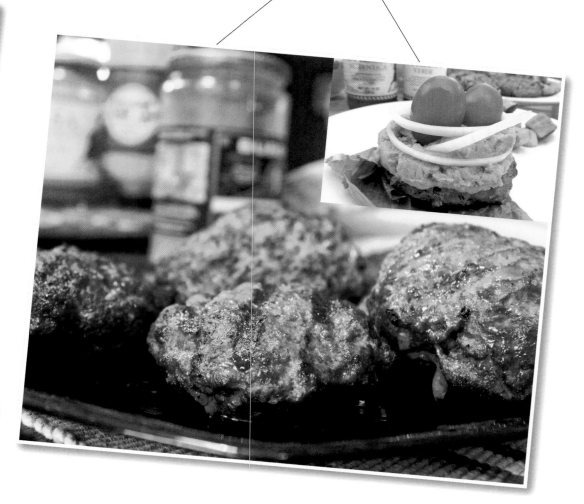

Special Tools:
Meat grinder or
food processor

Notes:

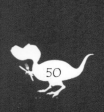

50

50/50 BACON BURGERS

Makes 6 burgers

You like bacon, right? How about bacon on hamburgers? Well, of course. They are delicious together! How about instead of putting the bacon on top of the burger, you put it in the burger? Mixing these two different meats together will be an opportunity to see how their textures feel and taste. Just be careful when making the patties; the more gentle your hands, the more juicy your hamburgers will be!

When we make burgers we love to "build our own." We often set out more than just the standard lettuce, tomato, and onion—we include things like guacamole and salsa, fried eggs, sautéed spinach, sauerkraut, and even roasted red peppers. We make special designs to see who can make us laugh the most. Our dino egg nest has been our favorite, but use your imagination. Use the burger as a base for whatever seems fun!

INGREDIENTS

⋄ 1 lb bacon	⋄ 1 tsp ground pepper
⋄ 1 lb lean ground red meat	⋄ 1 tsp paprika
⋄ 1½ tsp cumin	⋄ ½ tsp red pepper flakes (optional)

INSTRUCTIONS AND HOW KIDS CAN HELP

1. Grind the bacon with a meat grinder or chop with a food processor until the consistency is that of coarsely ground beef (ground bacon will feel slimy due to the high fat content).

2. Mix the ground meats with the spices by hand.

3. Form into 6 equal wide, 1-inch-thick patties (don't worry if they look a little big; the fat will drain out and shrink them more than normal beef burgers).

4. Grill, or cook on stovetop over medium heat to desired doneness, about 8 minutes per side.

5. Serve on a bed of lettuce with tomatoes for your own BLT, but Finian would tell you no burger is finished without guacamole.

Preheat grill to low or oven to 350 degrees

Notes:

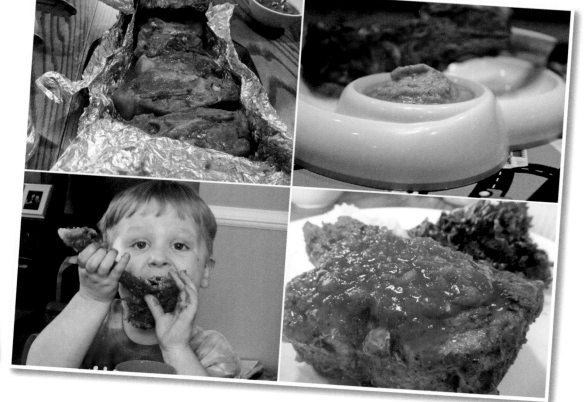

52

SHAKEY PORK BARBECUE

Serves 6

Have you ever heard of eating backbone? We hadn't either until we starting getting our meat from a very special farm called Polyface. They offer this awesome cut of meat that comes from the bone bumps along the back of a pig. Trust us—those pigs have some really delicious and tender back bones! Eating these bones is like living in a Flintstones cartoon—they're super big and tasty.

The meat tastes just like pork spare ribs, only the bone is shaped like a "T" or an "I" and there's more meat on each bone! This is the tastiest way we've learned to make it. If you can't find backbone where you live, you can use the same recipe to make delicious ribs, too. And don't forget to try it with our Texas Barbeque Sauce (p. 145)

INGREDIENTS

◇ 2 garlic cloves, minced	◇ 1 tsp paprika
◇ 1 Tbsp salt	◇ 1 tsp lemon zest
◇ 1 Tbsp unrefined granulated sugar (optional)	◇ pinch of cayenne
◇ 1 tsp black pepper	◇ 4 lbs pork backbone pieces (also called country ribs)

INSTRUCTIONS AND HOW KIDS CAN HELP

1. Combine spices in a plastic bag; add meat to bag.

2. Shake the bag until the spice mixture is rubbed over all of the meat.

3. Transfer the meat to a tinfoil pouch (we just wrap ours, but they make them specifically for this application).

4. Grill spice-rubbed meat in foil pouch over low heat in closed grill for 90 minutes or roast in oven at 350 degrees for 60 minutes (less if using ribs instead of back bone).

5. Increase heat to medium on grill and finish each cooked backbone by searing on both sides for about 2 minutes.

Main Dishes

Preheat half of the grill burners to low.
Soak wood chips in water for at least 30 minutes.

Special Tools: Wood chips for smoking. Meat thermometer is helpful.

Notes:

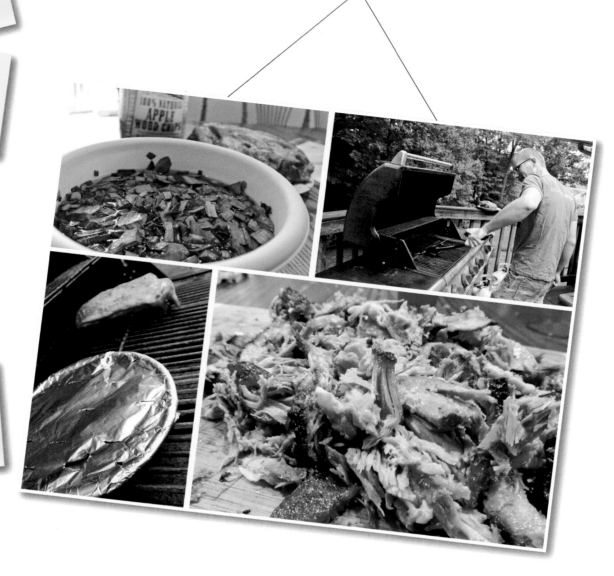

54

PULLED PORK

Serves 2 people per pound

When people think barbecue, they usually think pulled pork. It sounds hard to do, though; most people think they can't cook it at home. Well, as one of our favorite foods we wanted to figure out how to do it at home. And so we did, with just a plain ordinary gas grill! It was fun to learn about the different cuts of pork while looking into doing this ourselves. Did you know they call a pig's shoulder either "picnic" or "Boston butt"?

We dare you to give this a try and not like it. The pork is tender and juicy, while the skin remains nice and crisp. It's a perfect party food, too—sure to impress all your guests! We'd love for you to feel as awesome as we did when we made something that tasted as good as you can get at a restaurant with a pig on the sign. It's even better with our Texas Barbeque Sauce (p. 145)

INGREDIENTS

◇ 1 Tbsp salt	◇ ¼ tsp pepper
◇ 1 tsp paprika	◇ 2 tsp unrefined cane sugar (optional)
◇ 1 tsp garlic powder	◇ 6–10 lb pork shoulder, bone-in is best
◇ ½ tsp ground dry mustard	◇ 1½ C olive oil
◇ ½ tsp cumin	◇ ½ C apple cider vinegar

INSTRUCTIONS AND HOW KIDS CAN HELP

1. Combine all spices and sugar in small bowl with a fork.
2. Rub mixture over the shoulder, applying on all sides.
3. Add two handfuls of soaked chips to metal pie pan or baking dish, cover with foil and poke about a dozen ventilation holes in foil with a fork.
4. Place pie pan on heated side of the grill and shoulder on unheated side, close lid.
5. Mix together olive oil and vinegar.
6. Each hour, baste the shoulder with the oil and vinegar mixture to keep it moist.
7. Smoking will take about one hour per pound of shoulder or until the internal temperature reaches 190 degrees.
8. When finished cooking, pull pork apart with forks.

Main Dishes

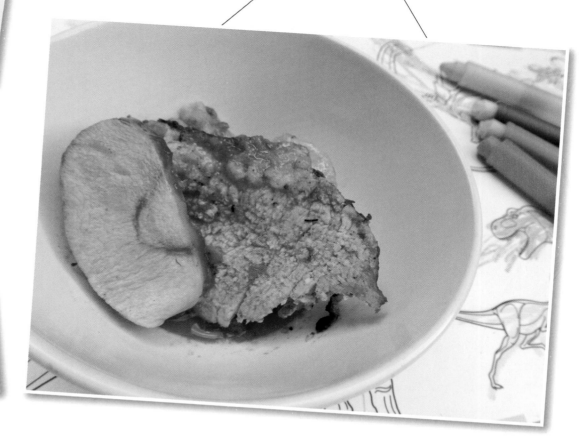

Preheat oven to
350 degrees

Special Tools:
Meat thermometer
is helpful

Notes:

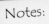
56

PORK ROAST WITH SQUISHY SQUASHY APPLES

Serves 6

The best thing about cooking a pork roast this way is that the juices from the pork ooze out and flavor the apples, making squashy apples you just won't be able to get enough of! The apples become salty and squishy like a pork-flavored applesauce. Delicious!

INGREDIENTS

- 1 clove garlic, minced
- 1 Tbsp salt
- 1 tsp paprika
- 1/2 tsp chili powder
- 1/2 tsp cinnamon
- 1/8 tsp ground cloves
- 3 lb pork roast, tied
- 6 apples, peeled, cored, and sliced into eighths

INSTRUCTIONS AND HOW KIDS CAN HELP

1. In a small bowl, combine spices into a rub using a fork.
2. Place roast in baking dish and rub spices on all sides.
3. Spread apples around roast in the dish.
4. Roast in oven at 350 degrees for 45–50 minutes until roast reaches 160 degrees.
5. Let meat rest 10 minutes before slicing.

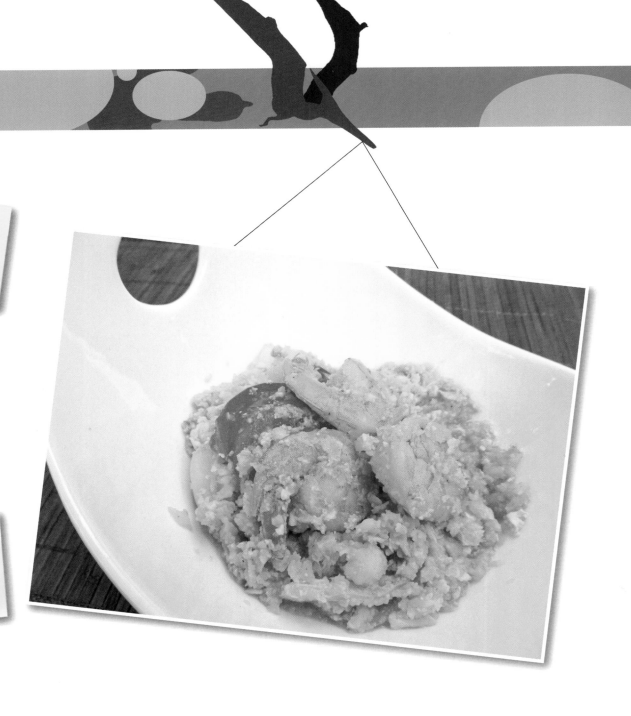

Special Tools:
Large wok or frying pan. Food processor. Microwave (optional, steaming would work as well).

Notes:

58

Fried Cauli Rice with Shrimp

Serves 4–6

Fried rice used to be a favorite in our house, but we don't eat rice anymore. Luckily, instead of rice you can use cauliflower. Once you have rice, you might as well fry it! The cauliflower rice is just as tasty as anything you could get delivered by a Chinese restaurant, so we like to serve ours on Friday nights before we watch a family movie or play games.

INGREDIENTS

- 1 head of cauliflower
- 1 Tbsp salt
- 2 Tbsp olive oil or lard
- 2 garlic cloves, minced
- 1 lb shrimp, peeled to the tail
- 1 onion, cut into 8 wedges
- 1 small tomato, cut into 8 wedges
- 2 eggs
- 1½ Tbsp fish sauce
- 1½ Tbsp coconut aminos
- ½ tsp ground pepper

INSTRUCTIONS AND HOW KIDS CAN HELP

1. Pulse cauliflower into rice-sized pieces in food processor.
2. Microwave cauliflower for three minutes.

Ta-da! This is the recipe for Cauliflower Rice!

3. Sprinkle rice with 1 Tbsp salt and set aside for at least 15 minutes.
4. Strain out excess water from cauliflower with colander, strainer, or cheesecloth.
5. Heat oil (or lard) over medium-high heat in a wok or large pan, cook garlic for a minute until it starts to brown.
6. Add shrimp, onion, and tomato and stir for two minutes.
7. Create an empty space in middle of wok (about a 4-inch-diameter void) and crack eggs into it; stir to scramble.
8. When egg is cooked, add cauliflower rice and keep stirring until everything is heated through and shrimp is pink on all sides.
9. Add fish sauce, aminos, and pepper and stir to combine before removing from heat.

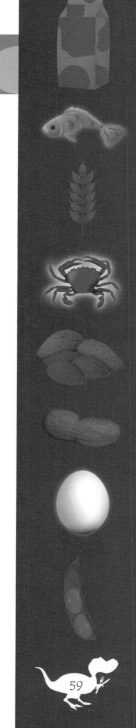

Main Dishes

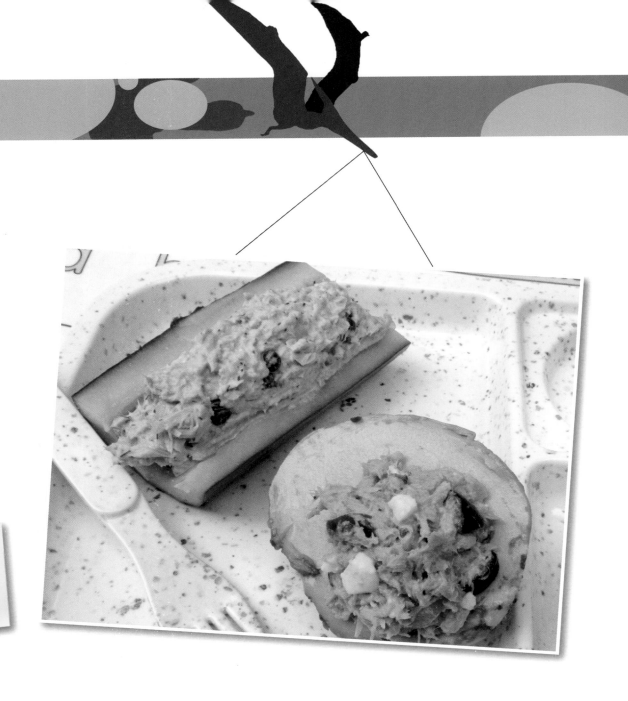

Notes:

60

FISH IN A BOAT AND COLE'S SALMON SALAD

Serves 4

When we make a "fish salad," either with tuna or salmon, we always put it in a veggie boat. We imagine that it's like the fish jumped out of the ocean and into a boat, no fishing pole required!

Our boys started taking these salads for lunch after Cole noticed that his mom was taking them for her lunch. He got so jealous he insisted we pack it for him, too. All of his teachers and classmates were impressed by his yummy lunch and some started bringing it for their lunch as well!

FISH IN A BOAT

- 1 (10 oz) can of chunk tuna, drained
- 1 carrot, peeled and grated
- ¼ C black olives, diced
- 1 hard-boiled egg, diced
- ⅓ C Mayonnaise (p. 137)
- 1 Tbsp pickle relish
- 1 Tbsp Dijon mustard
- 2 tsp salt
- dash of pepper

1. Place drained tuna in a bowl and break up with a fork.
2. Mix in carrot, olives, and egg until evenly mixed.
3. Add mayonnaise, relish, mustard, salt, and pepper.
4. Mix until combined.
5. Spoon into the boat of your choice!

COLE'S SALMON SALAD

- 1 (14.75 oz) can of boneless, skinless, wild-caught salmon
- ¼ C Lemon Dill Mayoli (p. 137)
- ¼ C capers, drained
- 2 tsp Dijon mustard
- pinch of salt
- dash of pepper

1. Place drained salmon in a bowl and break up with a fork.
2. Add Mayoli, capers, mustard, salt, and pepper.
3. Mix until combined.
4. Spoon into the boat of your choice!

61

Notes:

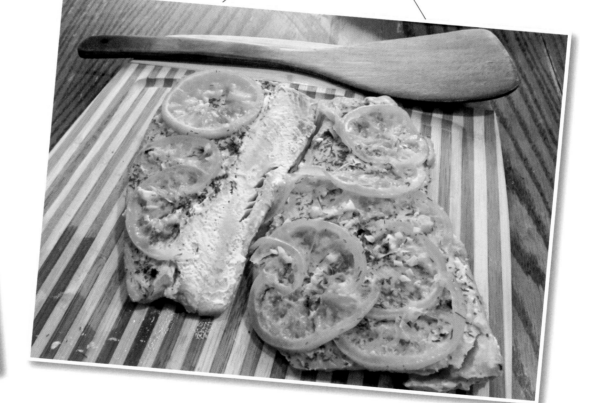

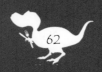
Eat Like a Dinosaur

Lemon Dill Salmon

Serves 6–8

Some kids think that they don't like to eat fish. We understand why: we've had fish we didn't like before, too. But if you try it when it's been cooked just right, you won't be able to resist it! Plus, salmon is super-good for you—it helps your entire body get into harmony with a special type of fat called Omega 3. It's also the kind of fat that helps your brain learn easily, so it's a great food to have the day before a test at school!

If you like this recipe, give our easy recipe, Cole's Salmon Salad (p. 61), a try too.

Ingredients

- 1 whole salmon filet, cut in two
- 3 cloves garlic, minced
- 1 Tbsp dill, fresh or dry
- salt and pepper
- 1 lemon, sliced $\frac{1}{8}$-inch thick rounds

Instructions and How Kids Can Help

 1. On a sheet of foil large enough to enclose, lay your filets down.

 2. Rub garlic, dill, salt, and pepper gently into flesh of salmon.

3. Lay sliced lemon rounds and cover top of filet.

4. Fold and enclose salmon in foil, grill or bake for 15–20 minutes.

5. Open carefully.

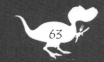

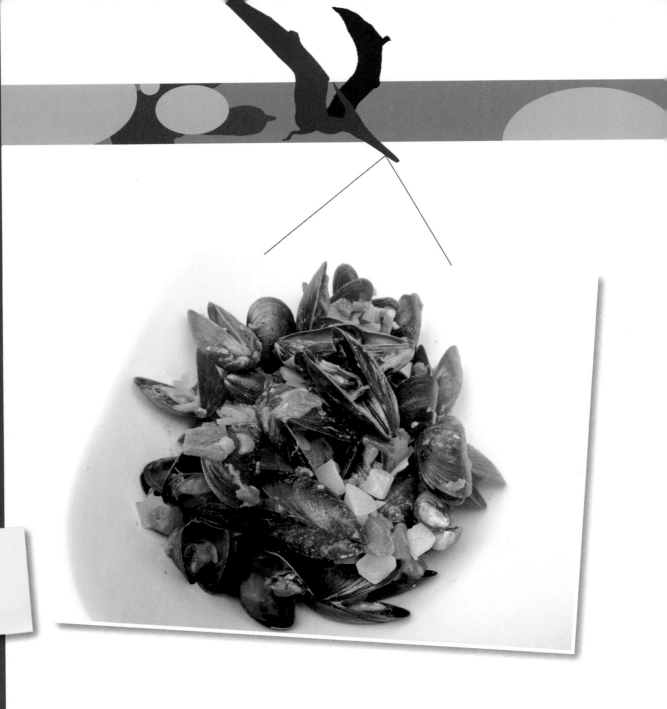

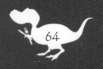

CURRIED MUSSELS, NOT MUSCLES

Serves 6

Mussels are not like the muscles in your body that make you strong. They're little creatures inside black shells that cling to rocks in the ocean. When you get them from the store, they are still alive (be careful and use gentle hands)! When you prepare them for cooking they'll open and close their shells as you wash them. You also have to remove their beard, which is the part of their body that allow them to cling on to the rocks where they live.

When you put the mussels in the hot pot, you are able to watch them go from moving around to being ready to eat. When they're cooked, their shells open up, and we like to make their shells flap open and closed and pretend they talk to each other—what do your mussels say?

INGREDIENTS

⋄ 2½ lbs mussels	⋄ 1 Tbsp garlic powder
⋄ 2 Tbsp olive oil	⋄ 2 Tbsp yellow curry powder
⋄ 2 medium yellow onions, diced	⋄ 1 (14 oz) can full-fat coconut milk
⋄ 2 (14 oz) cans diced tomatoes	⋄ 1 C water

INSTRUCTIONS AND HOW KIDS CAN HELP

1. To clean mussels, wash and scrub the outside of their shells and pull off any remaining stringy "beard" from the hinged side of the shell; inspect for broken shells and throw those away.
2. Heat oil over medium in a pot and add onions; cook until soft, about 6 minutes.
3. Add tomatoes, garlic, and curry powder to pot and stir.
4. Add coconut milk and water and bring to a soft boil on medium heat.
5. Add mussels, stir and toss to coat in sauce, and cover for 8 minutes.
6. When done, all shells should have opened and meat should easily pop out of shell.

Main Dishes

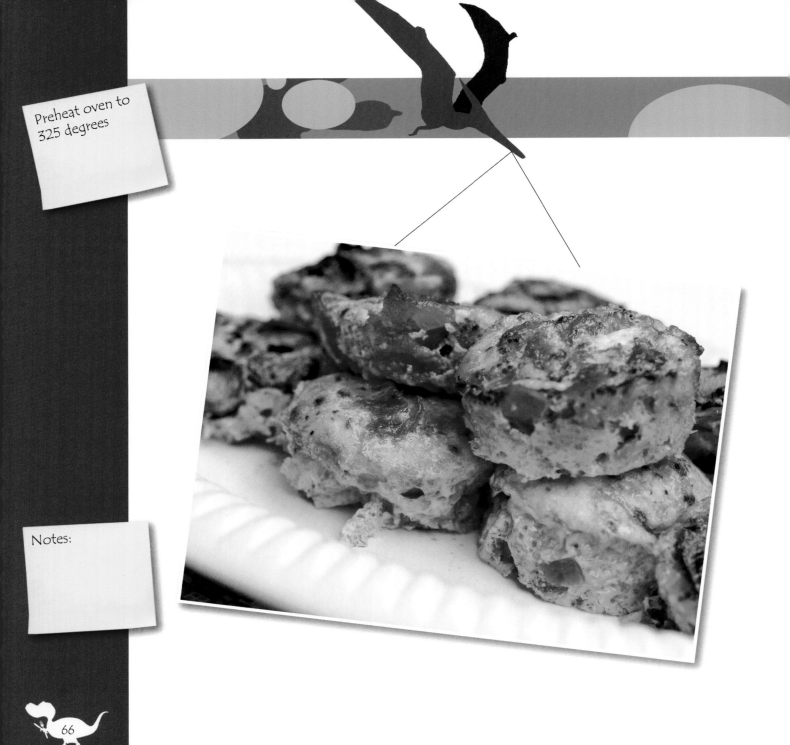

Eat Like a Dinosaur

MINI EGG PIZZAS

Makes 20 egg cups

When we make egg muffins we like to make up silly names like Lady Gaga's Egg Cups. This variation might not be as silly, but we know exactly why it's called *Mini Egg Pizzas*—because it tastes like pizza! When we make these, we put sliced black olives (Cole's favorite) in half the batch and chopped mushrooms (Finian's favorite) in the other half so that it really tastes like their favorite pizza. Add your favorite pizza toppings to these muffins, and you can have your favorite pizza for breakfast!

On Sundays we make a whole bunch of these so we have them all week. You could do that too. Just stick them in the freezer and microwave yourself an egg muffin on your way to the bus stop. Pizza for breakfast. How awesome is that?

INGREDIENTS

- 1 Tbsp olive oil or lard
- 1 small red onion, diced
- 1 Tbsp tomato paste
- 1 (14 oz) can diced tomatoes, strained
- 1 C nitrate-free pepperoni, diced
- 10 eggs
- 1 tsp dried oregano
- 1 tsp dried basil
- 1 tsp salt
- ¼ tsp black pepper
- ½ C black olives, chopped (optional)
- ½ C mushrooms, chopped (optional)

INSTRUCTIONS AND HOW KIDS CAN HELP

1. Heat olive oil or lard in medium frying pan over medium heat.
2. Sauté onions until almost softened, about 5 minutes.
3. Add tomato paste to pan, cook and stir for one minute until well incorporated with onions.
4. Add tomatoes; cook 2 minutes, stirring frequently.
5. Add pepperoni; cook together for 4 minutes, stirring frequently. Set aside.
6. Crack and beat eggs in a bowl.
7. Add oregano, basil, salt, and pepper to eggs and mix.
8. Spoon 1 Tbsp of tomato mixture plus any other toppings into each greased or lined muffin cup.
9. Ladle egg mixture into muffin cups until they are ¾ full (eggs do fluff up in oven).
10. Bake at 325 degrees for 20 minutes until cooked through and eggs brown slightly on top.

Main Dishes

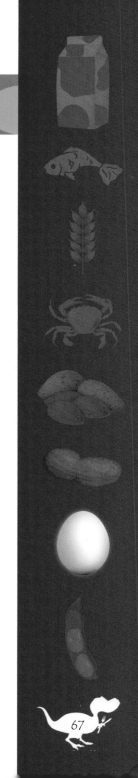

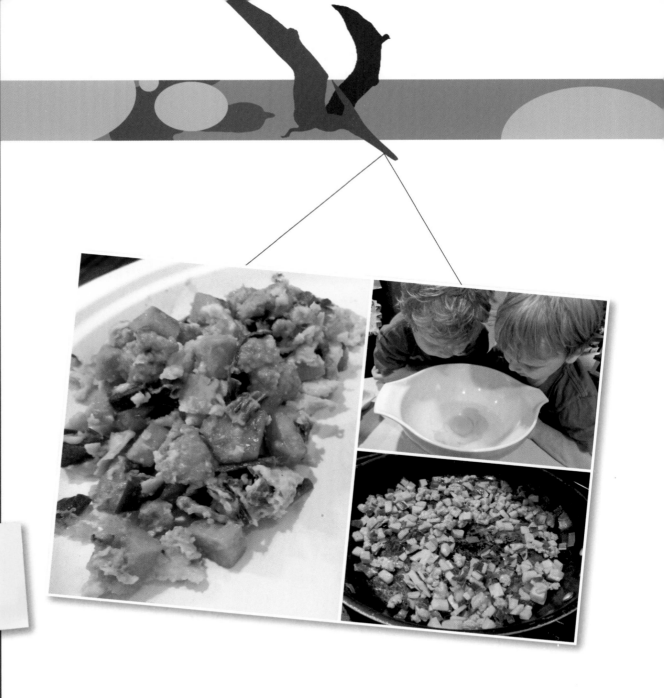

Notes:

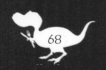

Eat Like a Dinosaur

GOOSE EGG SCRAMBLE

Serves 4

Goose and duck eggs have large, nutrient-rich egg yolks. Did you know they are a wonderful combination of fat, protein, vitamins, and minerals that your body loves to absorb to help your body and brain grow? When we found goose eggs at our local farmers' market, we talked about how they might be different from our usual chicken eggs. Immediately our boys insisted we try them!

We learned that the larger the egg, the harder it is to crack. If goose eggs took a lot of muscle to crack, what would an Ostrich egg take? A hammer?

INGREDIENTS

- 1 lb nitrate-free pork breakfast sausage
- 2 medium sweet potatoes, peeled and diced
- 2 scallions (we use the onion greens growing in our garden), sliced
- 2 goose eggs (4 duck eggs or 6 chicken eggs)

INSTRUCTIONS AND HOW KIDS CAN HELP

1. Sauté sausage and sweet potatoes over medium heat until potatoes are soft, about 10 minutes; if your sausage is not fatty enough, add a tablespoon or two of the fat of your choice.

2. Add scallions once sausage is brown and sweet potatoes are cooked through.

3. While waiting for mixture to cook, crack and scramble eggs, making sure to add lots of airy bubbles.

4. Pour eggs over sausage, potato, and onion mixture, stirring continuously.

5. Cook until eggs are done (about 5 minutes).

Main Dishes

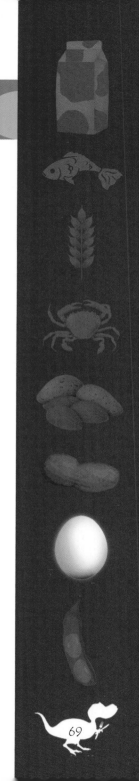

Notes:

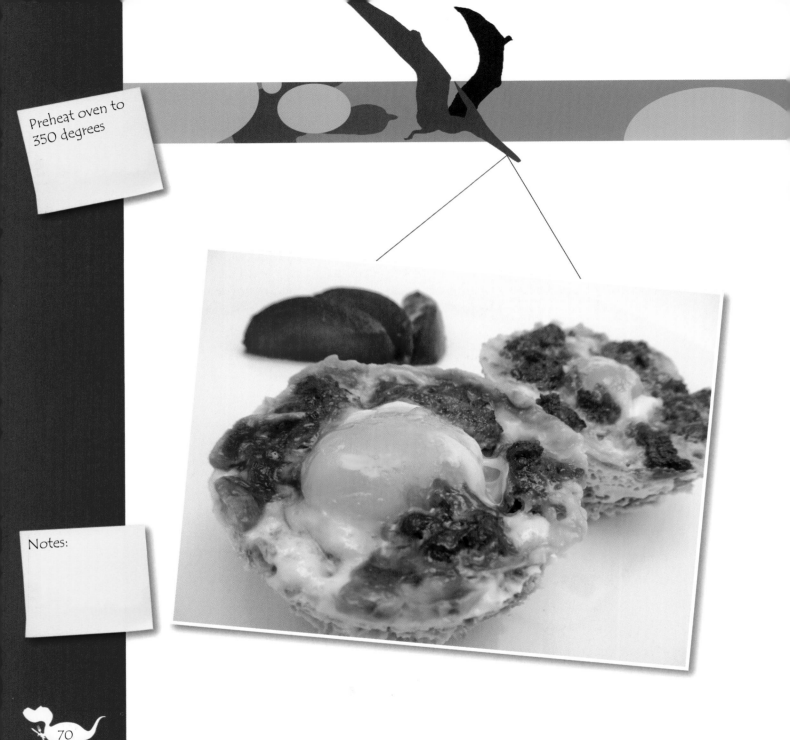

70

EGGS IN A NEST

Makes 12 "nests"

When Stacy was growing up, Sundays were a day when her mom made special breakfasts. Often it was the same breakfast Stacy's mom had asked for when she was a kid: an "egg in a nest." Back then, the nest was a piece of toast, pan fried, with the center torn out. Drop the egg into the hole and, voila—an egg in a nest!

The egg nests were a fun breakfast that we all missed, so we thought we'd use a slightly different approach to make our own eggs in nests. Since sausage tastes better than toast, it is a nice replacement. Best of all, you can bake a big batch of these little nests in advance and have them available and ready to reheat early in the mornings without any effort at all!

INGREDIENTS

- ½ lb nitrate-free breakfast sausage, loose
- 12 medium eggs
- 2 Tbsp olive oil

INSTRUCTIONS AND HOW KIDS CAN HELP

1. Thoroughly grease muffin tin or use silicone muffin pan.

2. Use a heaping spoon of sausage to make a nest on the outside edges of the muffin tin—use a thin layer around the edges so that there is room to drop in the egg. We recommend making one complete nest with an egg first before lining the rest to ensure you have enough space for the egg.

3. Open eggs one at a time and drop carefully into each lined egg cup.

4. Drizzle top of each egg with olive oil.

5. Bake at 350 degrees for 23–28 minutes, until eggs are cooked to your liking.

6. Let nests cool about 5 minutes, release the edges of the nests with a butter knife and pop them out.

Main Dishes

71

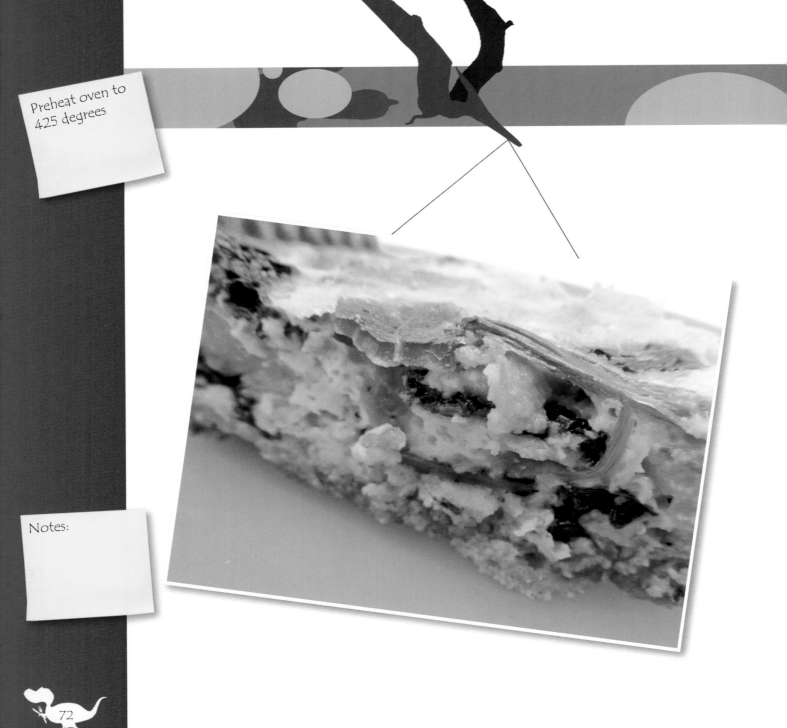

Preheat oven to 425 degrees

Notes:

Eat Like a Dinosaur

SWEET QUICHE

Serves 6-8

Another name for this could be the Italian flag egg pie because it's got red bacon, white apples, and green spinach—and it's a pie. Egg pies, also known as quiches, are a fun way to eat your eggs. If you'd like, you can find different ways to make this for yourself. Try broccoli instead of spinach or perhaps ham cubes instead of bacon. Anyway you put it together it will be delicious!

INGREDIENTS

- ⅓ lb nitrate-free bacon, diced
- 2 apples, peeled and diced
- ½ tsp cumin
- 2 C spinach
- 4 eggs
- ½ C full-fat canned coconut milk
- ½ tsp salt
- ⅛ tsp pepper
- 1 prebaked pie crust (p. 207) (optional)

INSTRUCTIONS AND HOW KIDS CAN HELP

1. Sauté chopped bacon over medium-high heat until fat begins to render, about 3 minutes.

2. Turn heat to medium and add apples and cumin to bacon.

3. Cook and stir occasionally until apples soften, about 5 minutes.

4. Add spinach and keep tossing until it begins to wilt, about 2 minutes—remove from heat and let cool for 5–10 minutes.

5. In a bowl combine eggs, coconut milk, salt, and pepper—whisk until bubbly.

6. Lay vegetable mixture into precooked pie crust if using, or greased pie pan if not.

7. Pour egg mixture over vegetables.

8. Cover edges of pie crust with aluminum foil or pie crust protector.

9. Bake for 15 minutes at 425 degrees, then turn oven down to 300 degrees and bake for 30 minutes.

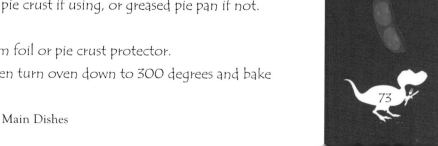

Preheat oven to
350 degrees

Notes:

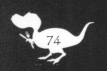

74

Eat Like a Dinosaur

Kale, Bacon, & Black Olive Egg Pie

Serves 6–10 slices

Sometimes for breakfast we make egg pies, otherwise known as frittatas. If you used a crust, it'd be called a quiche. No matter what you call this recipe, it's super-delicious. The kale gets crispy on the top and adds a nice crunch! It's best hot, but sometimes we steal leftover pieces right out of the fridge as we're running out the door!

Kale is a fantastic vegetable we think everyone should try. It's a crinkly leaf that's kind of purplish-green and is full of great vitamins and minerals. And then we add two other favorites, black olives and bacon, to make this super yummy. We have it for breakfast, lunch, and dinner.

INGREDIENTS

- ⅓ lb nitrate-free bacon
- 2 C kale, chopped
- 1 C black olives, chopped
- 8 eggs
- ¼ tsp black pepper
- 1 prebaked pie crust (p. 207) (optional)

INSTRUCTIONS AND HOW KIDS CAN HELP

1. Cook bacon in frying pan over medium heat until crispy, about 10 minutes.
2. Remove bacon from the pan and crumble when cooled.
3. Add kale to pan with bacon fat, tossing frequently; cook until softened, about 3 minutes (do not allow to wilt entirely; it will cook more in the pie).
4. Add crumbled bacon and olives to pan with kale, cook 2 minutes until warmed through and well combined.
5. Lay vegetable mixture into precooked pie crust if using, or greased pie pan if not.
6. Beat eggs in bowl with pepper.
7. Pour egg mixture over vegetables.
8. Cover edges of pie crust with aluminum foil or pie crust protector.
9. Bake in 350-degree oven for 25–30 minutes; remove once the top becomes a light golden brown.

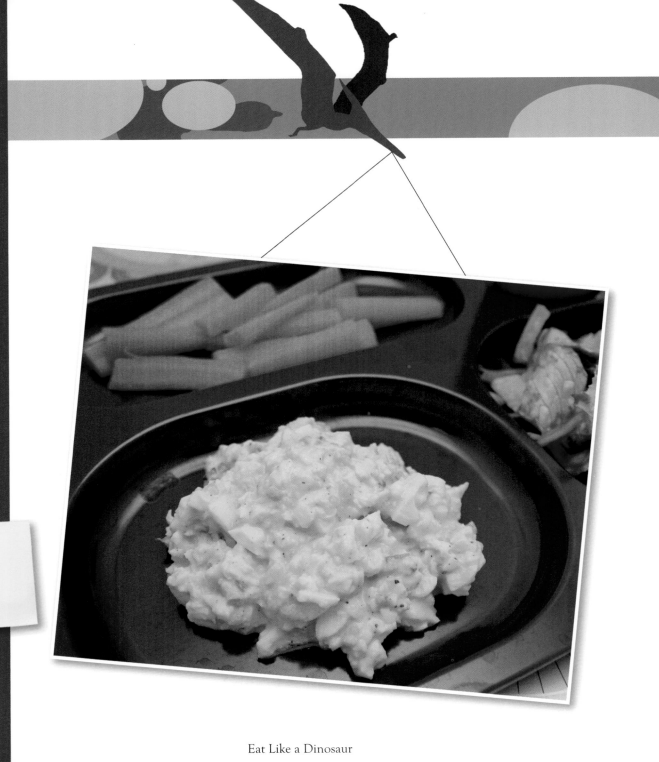

Notes:

76

Egg Salad

Serves 4

One of the members of our family had never even heard of egg salad (if you were here with us you could see us pointing at Matt). Now he loves how quick it is to make, and delicious too! It's so easy, and kids can help with every step; Cole even makes it by himself sometimes. Eggs, pickles, and mayonnaise—what's not to love?

Finian (of course) loves to use an avocado as his egg salad boat, but Cole likes to eat egg salad with tomatoes. We think you should try a lettuce boat with a slice of bacon and tomatoes. Mmmm . . . yum!

INGREDIENTS

- 8 eggs, hard-boiled and peeled
- ½ C mayonnaise (p. 137)
- ⅓ C pickle relish (we recommend Bubbies brand)
- 1 tsp Dijon mustard
- ¼ tsp salt
- ¼ tsp pepper

INSTRUCTIONS AND HOW KIDS CAN HELP

 1. Slice or mash eggs to break up egg whites a bit.

 2. Add remaining ingredients to bowl.

 3. Stir and mash all ingredients together until thoroughly combined.

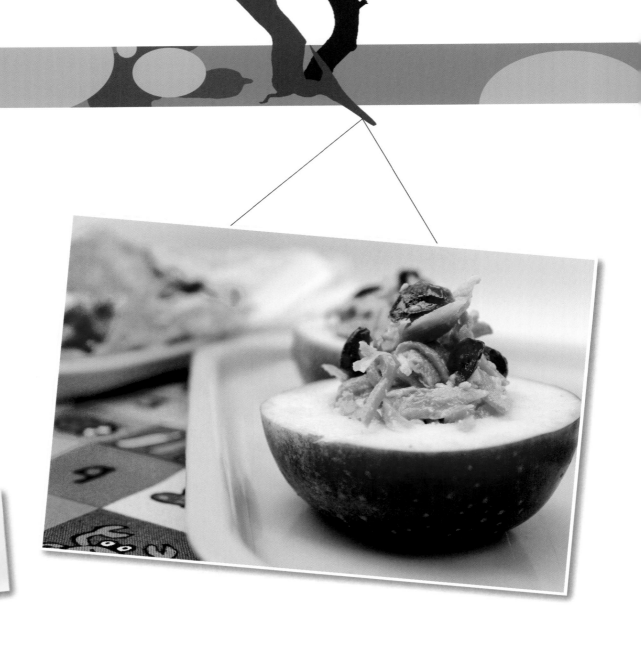

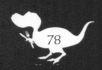

Notes:

Eat Like a Dinosaur

Maple Chicken Salad

Serves 4

Do you like maple syrup on your pancakes? Well then, you'll probably love it on your chicken! You might think it sounds weird, but we thought it sounded delicious . . . and you betcha it is!

You can use this salad to make boats just like the Fish in a Boat (p. 61). We think you'd like it if you put the salad in an apple boat! Just cut the apple in half, remove the core, and spoon your chicken in it! Our favorite way to eat Maple Chicken Salad is to put it on a romaine lettuce leaf because it's crispy, fresh, and able to hold lots of chicken!

If you use regular mayonnaise instead of our Bacon Mayonnaise (p. 137), consider adding some crumbled bacon into your salad—it really brings the flavors together.

INGREDIENTS

- 1 C chicken, cooked and shredded (you could use canned chicken breast, but this is a great recipe for leftover chicken)
- ¾ C carrot, shredded
- ¼ C dried cranberries
- 3 Tbsp Bacon Mayonnaise (p. 137)
- 1 Tbsp maple syrup
- pinch of salt
- dash of black pepper

INSTRUCTIONS AND HOW KIDS CAN HELP

 Mix together chicken, carrots, and cranberries.

 Add mayonnaise, syrup, salt (taste first, the bacon mayonnaise is already salty), and pepper.

 Mix until combined, and enjoy!

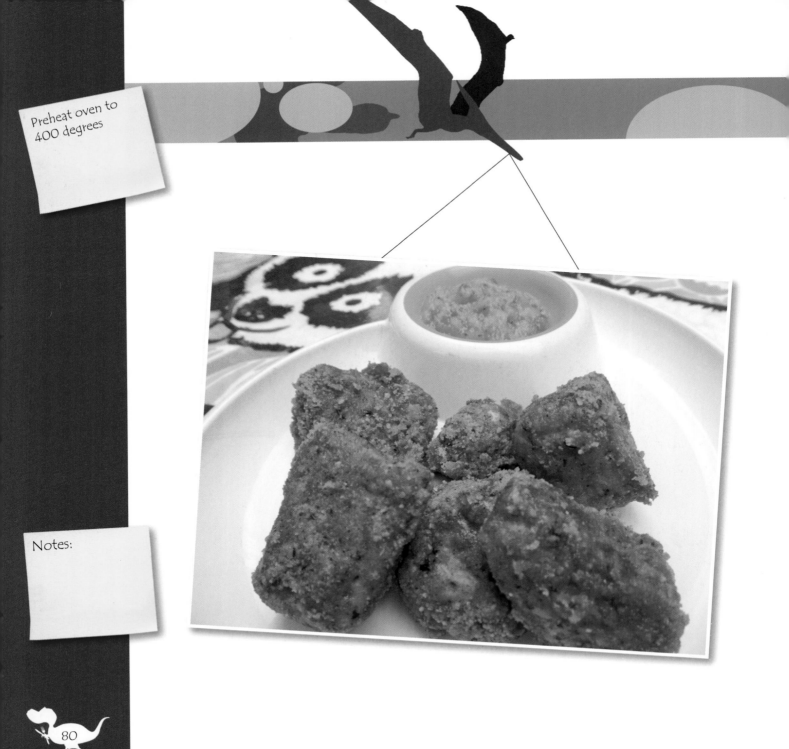

Notes:

80

Eat Like a Dinosaur

FOOL'S GOLD (CHICKEN NUGGETS)

Serves 4

One of the things our boys always want and miss is chicken nuggets. We went into our kitchen laboratory and came up with this fun way to make chicken nuggets with healthy ingredients so that their daydreams about nuggets could come true.

We like to keep a cooked batch in the freezer so that Uncle Andrew has something easy to heat up for the boys when he babysits. We love these with our Southwestern Pineapple Sauce (p. 149).

INGREDIENTS

- 3 chicken breasts, deboned and skinned
- 2 C almond flour
- 2 Tbsp arrowroot powder
- 2 tsp salt
- 1 tsp paprika
- 1 tsp onion powder
- ½ tsp dry mustard
- ⅛ tsp black pepper
- ¾ C olive oil

INSTRUCTIONS AND HOW KIDS CAN HELP

1. Cut chicken into 1-inch by 1-inch chunks.
2. Mix flour, arrowroot powder, and spices together in bowl with a fork or whisk.
3. Pour olive oil into a separate bowl.
4. Dip each chicken piece in the oil and then roll in the flour mixture.
5. Place nuggets on baking sheet and bake for 15–20 minutes at 400 degrees, flipping halfway through.
6. When done, the crust will be golden brown and juices will run clear.

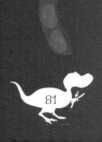

Preheat oven to 375 degrees

Special Tools: Wire rack for cookie sheets (we use our cookie cooling racks)

Notes:

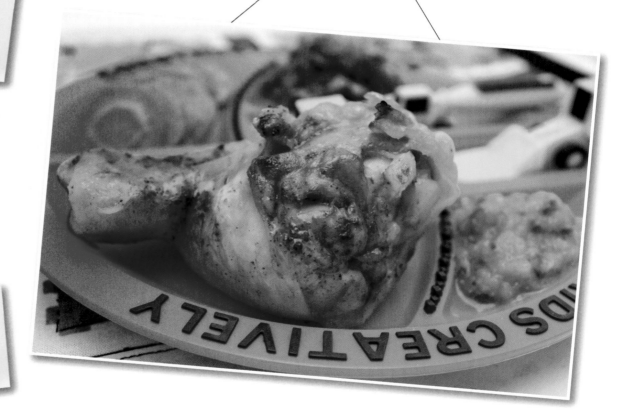

82

HISSIN' CHICKEN

Serves 4

When you roast chicken in the oven, you can actually hear it talking to you! As it cooks, chicken will hiss and crackle the entire time. We love to double this recipe so that we have enough chicken to take for lunch the next day. Stacy's family is from Hungary, so we like the spice paprika. If you don't like paprika, use a little pepper instead or have fun choosing the seasoning of your choice.

INGREDIENTS

- ⋄ 6 chicken legs or 4 chicken thighs (about 2 ½ lbs)
- ⋄ 2 Tbsp melted coconut oil or lard
- ⋄ 1 tsp salt
- ⋄ 1 tsp paprika

INSTRUCTIONS AND HOW KIDS CAN HELP

 Pat chicken thighs dry with a towel.

 Place chicken on wire rack, set into a baking sheet.

Sprinkle chicken with oil, salt, and paprika; rub chicken to thoroughly coat.

4. Roast at 375 degrees for 45 minutes until chicken is cooked through.

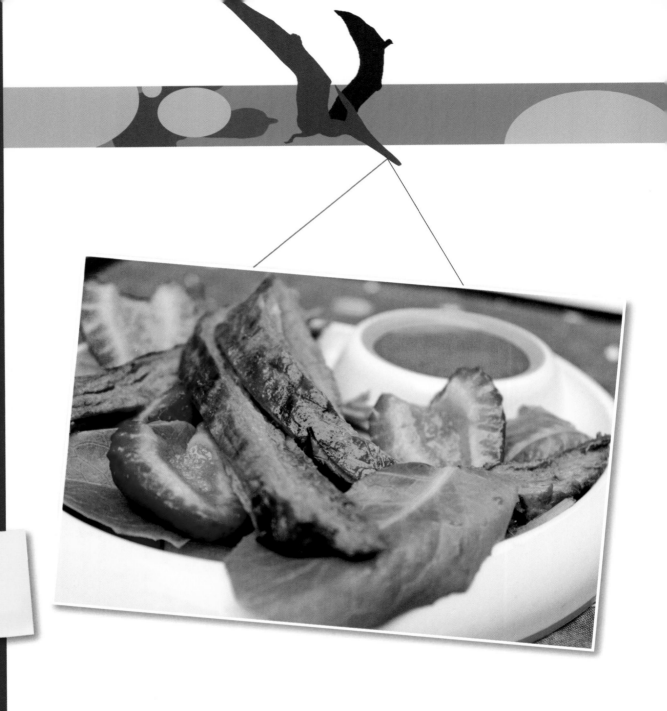

Eat Like a Dinosaur

Notes:

STEAK & STRAWBERRY SALAD

Serves 4

Sometimes the best way to eat a salad is to put a steak on it! It's the perfect "eat like a dinosaur" meal: both a T-Rex and a Triceratops could share it! This is one of our favorite dinners, and it will make you believe that salad can be delicious. We always ask for seconds. We recommend you eat it with our Raspberry Dressing (p. 147).

INGREDIENTS

- 1½ lb flank steak
- ½ tsp salt
- ¼ tsp pepper
- 4 C baby mixed greens
- 1 pt of strawberries, sliced
- 1 bell pepper, diced
- 1 carrot, sliced into rounds

INSTRUCTIONS AND HOW KIDS CAN HELP

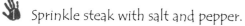 Sprinkle steak with salt and pepper.

2. Add room-temperature flank steak to hot pan and cook over medium-high heat about 6 minutes per side for medium rare.

3. Allow steak to rest uncovered for 10 minutes, slice steak into ½-inch strips on the bias.

Toss all ingredients, including meat.

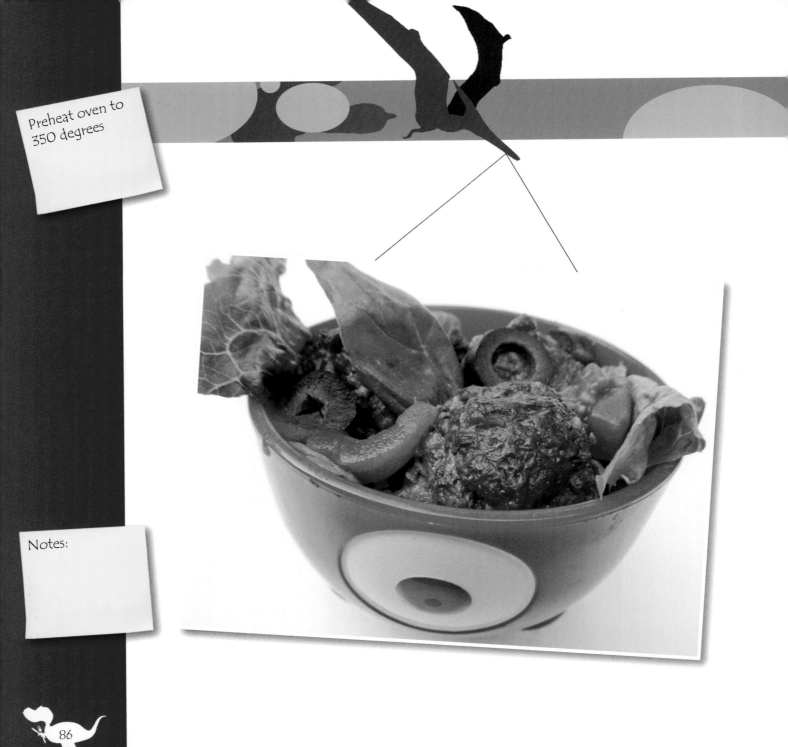

Eat Like a Dinosaur

MEATBALL SALAD

Serves 4

What happens if you take the bread and pasta out of a big spaghetti dinner? You're left with meatballs and salad. And since we like meatballs on everything, we thought maybe a meatball salad might be tasty. We hope you like our idea, too!

This is a fun and different way to eat meatballs that we really enjoy. Eating them this way has all the flavors of great Italian food in a healthful salad!

INGREDIENTS

- 1 lb ground red meat
- 1 egg
- ½ tsp dried oregano
- ½ tsp salt
- ⅛ tsp ground pepper
- 12 basil leaves, sliced thinly
- 1 heart of romaine in 1-inch ribbons
- 1 (14 oz) can diced tomatoes, drained
- ½ C sliced black olives, drained and rinsed
- 3 Tbsp balsamic vinegar

INSTRUCTIONS AND HOW KIDS CAN HELP

1. Combine beef, egg, oregano, salt, and pepper in a bowl; mix by hand until thoroughly combined.

2. Form mixture into 1½-inch meatballs (a heaping tablespoon) and place in 9-by-13-inch baking dish or baking sheet with a lip.

3. Bake in 350-degree oven for 15 minutes, until cooked through.

4. Toss meatballs with remaining ingredients of the salad, sprinkling the vinegar on top.

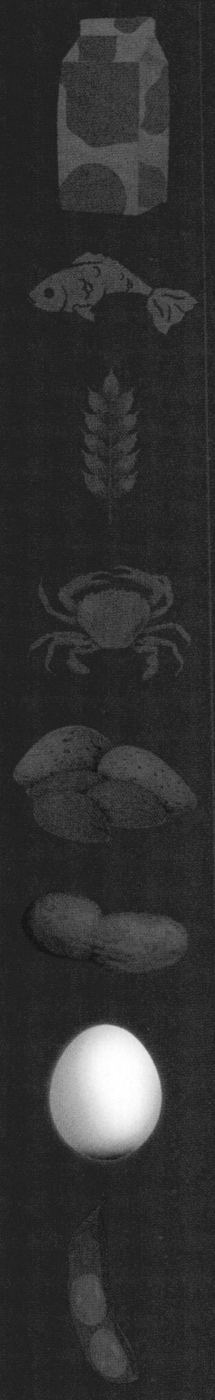

Main Dishes

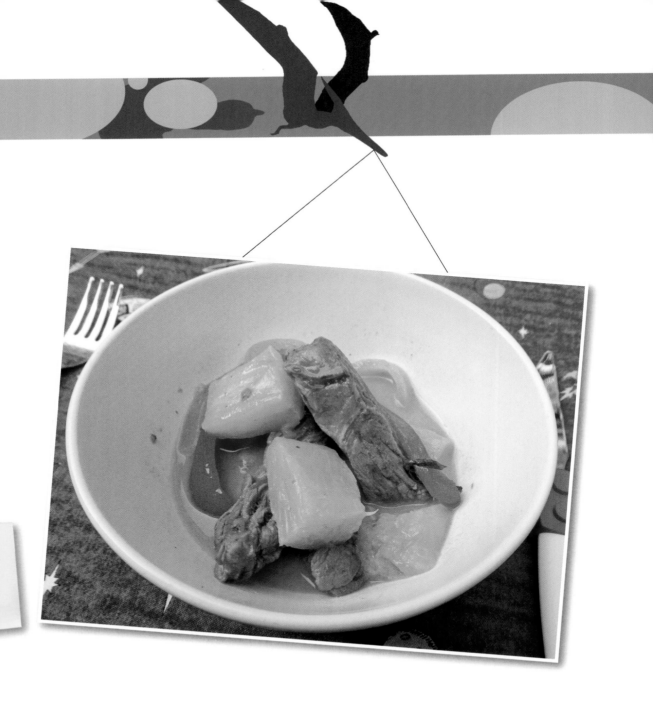

Notes:

88

Eat Like a Dinosaur

PINEAPPLE CURRY

Serves 6

When someone says "curry," what they mean is tasty spices mixed into a sauce with meat and veggies. This is a curry based on what they make in a country called Thailand, where coconut milk is used in curries. Often Thai curries are very spicy, but in this recipe the sweet pineapple makes a perfect complement to the rich coconut milk and beef!

If you use canned pineapple, like we usually do, make sure to get it in juice rather than syrup so you can make our Pineapple, Mint, and Clementine Water (p. 187).

INGREDIENTS

- 2 Tbsp coconut oil
- 2 lbs flank steak cut into ½-inch-by-2-inch strips
- 1 medium onion, sliced
- 1 red pepper, sliced

- 2 (14 oz) cans full-fat coconut milk
- 1 pineapple, cubed or 1 (20 oz) can of pineapple chunks
- 2 Tbsp red curry paste
- 1 Tbsp fish sauce

INSTRUCTIONS AND HOW KIDS CAN HELP

1. Melt coconut oil over medium heat in a large frying pan.
2. Add meat and brown on all sides, about 5 minutes; set aside.
3. Add sliced onions and peppers and cook until soft, about 8 minutes.
4. Add coconut milk, pineapple, curry paste, and fish sauce, stir to combine.
5. Return meat and accumulated juices to pan.
6. Reduce heat to low and cover, simmer for 20 minutes.
7. Serve over Cauliflower Rice (p. 59).

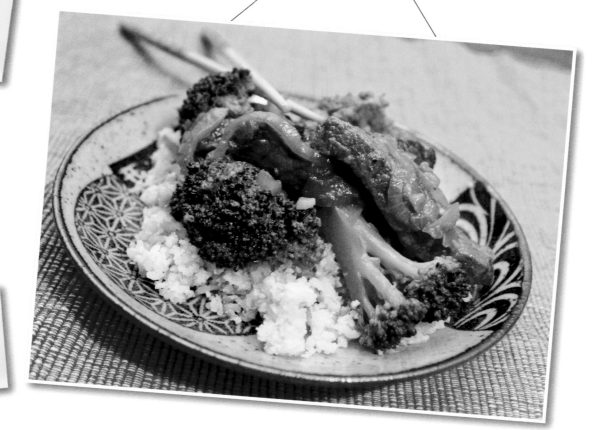

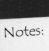

Eat Like a Dinosaur

BEEF & BROCCOLI

Serves 4–6

We LOVED to order Chinese takeout until we found out that there is a lot of wheat in the soy sauce. How silly is it to have wheat in your soy sauce? Rather than give up on eating Chinese food, we started making our own.

This beef and broccoli is a little bit sweet, just the right amount of salty, and is a very tasty version of one of our old favorites. Make it with our Fried Cauli Rice with Shrimp (p. 59) for the perfect "takeout" meal at home.

INGREDIENTS

- 1 lb sirloin steak, sliced into strips ½-inch by ½-inch by 2-inch
- 2 Tbsp olive oil or lard
- 1 medium onion, sliced
- 2 cloves of garlic, minced
- 1 lb broccoli, chopped into 2- to 3-inch pieces
- ¼ C coconut aminos (or wheat-free tamari)
- 2 tsp sesame oil
- 1 tsp salt
- ⅛ tsp pepper
- ⅛ tsp red pepper flakes

INSTRUCTIONS AND HOW KIDS CAN HELP

1. Heat large frying pan or wok over medium-high heat; if meat is lean, consider adding 1 Tbsp of oil to pan.
2. Sear beef for about 2 minutes on each side, then remove from pan and set aside.
3. Turn heat down to medium and add oil in wok to warm.
4. Add onions to wok, cooking and stirring with little hands until onions start to soften, about 5 minutes.
5. Add garlic and cooked meat to wok, allow to cook together for 3–4 minutes.
6. Add broccoli, aminos, sesame oil, salt, pepper, and red pepper flakes to pan.
7. Stir to combine, reduce heat to low and simmer for 30 minutes, covered.

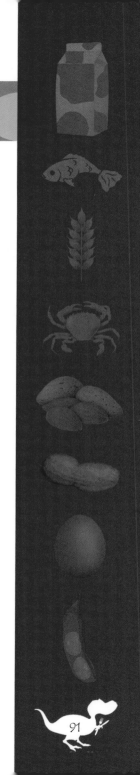

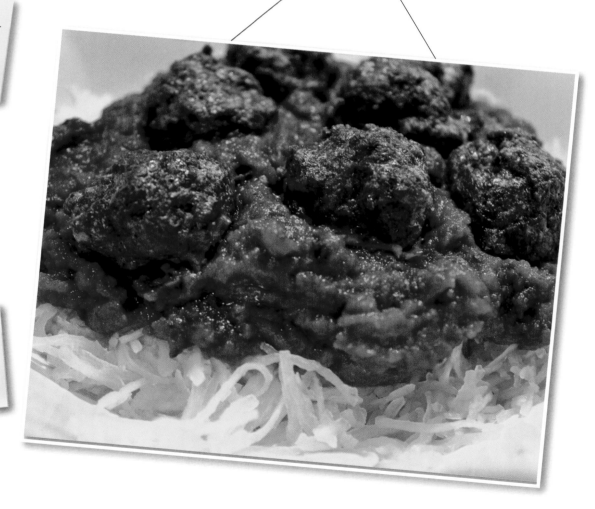

Special Tools:
Microwave (Alternatively, you can roast squash for 45 minutes at 350 degrees)

Notes:

92

Eat Like a Dinosaur

Spaghetti with Meatballs

Serves 6

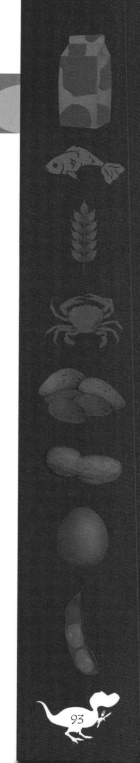

Did you get a little sad when you decided that you wouldn't be eating spaghetti anymore? We did, too. Stacy's grandmother is from Italy and her whole family loves spaghetti. They even call the sauce "gravy" because they like to put it on almost everything.

We were so happy when we tried a special vegetable that is MADE out of spaghetti! It's called a spaghetti squash, and it is yummy! Once you cook it, you scoop out the "noodles" and you have spaghetti once again!

INGREDIENTS

- 1 medium spaghetti squash, halved lengthwise
- 1 lb ground red meat
- 1 beef liver, ground or 1 egg
- 2 (14.5 oz) cans of diced tomatoes, drained and puréed
- 2 tsp salt

- 1 tsp black pepper
- 1 tsp dried oregano
- 1 tsp dried thyme
- 1 Tbsp apple cider or juice
- 1 Tbsp tomato paste
- 10 basil leaves, sliced

INSTRUCTIONS AND HOW KIDS CAN HELP

1. Microwave both halves of the squash on a plate cut side down about 10 minutes or until easily pierced with fork.
2. Scrape out the "noodles" from the squash into serving bowl.
3. Combine meats together by hand and roll into tablespoon-sized balls.
4. Bake meatballs in oven for 15 minutes at 350 degrees.
5. Over high heat add tomatoes, salt, pepper, oregano, thyme, and cider, into medium saucepan and let come to a boil—let little hands stir occasionally.
6. Decrease heat to low and add paste and basil—let little hands stir occasionally.
7. Cover tomato sauce and let simmer for 20 minutes.
8. Add cooked meatballs and sauce over the squash noodles.

Preheat oven to 275 degrees, then 350 degree

Special Tools: Meat grinder or food processor

Notes:

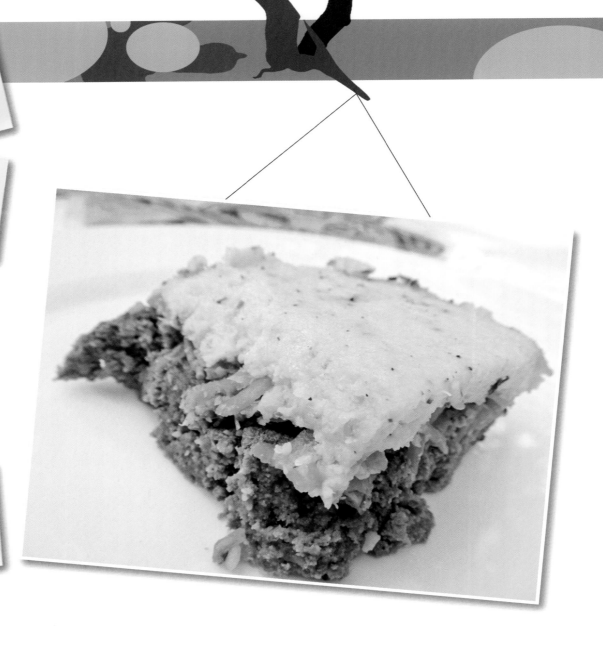

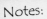 94

SHEPHERD'S PIE

Serves 6-8

Shepherd's Pie is a really famous dish that is made in the United Kingdom and other parts of Europe. It's in layers, just like lasagna; but, instead of pasta, there's a mash on top! In this recipe, we build a base of super-healthy meat from the organs of animals (make sure to check out that beef heart before you grind it up. It's really cool!). You may not have ever had organ meats before, but you should definitely try it out. Just like in our own bodies, animal organs have much more vitamins and minerals than the muscle meat you're used to eating. You could also try ground beef liver instead of heart for this recipe. We try to eat offal, or organ meat, at least once a week.

The best part of making this dish, which we also call Organ Meat Pie, is spreading all the layers over each other and then seeing them when you cut into the "pie" on your plate at dinnertime. It's like a little rainbow on your plate!

INGREDIENTS

◊ ¾ lb ground red meat, more if not using optional meats	◊ 1 head cauliflower, stems removed and chopped
◊ 1 beef heart, ground (optional)	◊ 1 tsp salt
◊ ½ lb lamb kidneys, cleaned and ground (optional)	◊ ½ tsp pepper
◊ 1 tsp salt	◊ ½ C carrot, shredded
◊ ½ tsp pepper	◊ ½ C celery, shredded
◊ 1 tsp cumin	◊ ½ C broccoli, shredded
◊ 1 tsp paprika	◊ 1 Tbsp fresh basil, chopped
	◊ 2 tsp fresh rosemary, chopped

INSTRUCTIONS AND HOW KIDS CAN HELP

1. Mix meats together with salt, pepper, cumin, and paprika.
2. Spread evenly in 9-by-13-inch pan and cook uncovered at 275 degrees for 30 minutes.
3. Steam cauliflower (covered in the microwave or over boiling water) for 10 minutes or until fork tender.
4. Purée cauliflower with food processor with salt and pepper. Set aside.
5. Mix shredded vegetables with basil and rosemary.
6. Spread uncooked, shredded vegetables over cooked meat.
7. Spread mashed cauliflower evenly over meat and vegetables.
8. Cook at 350 degrees for 45 minutes.

Main Dishes

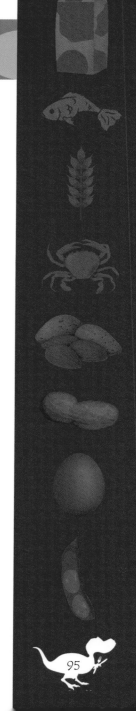

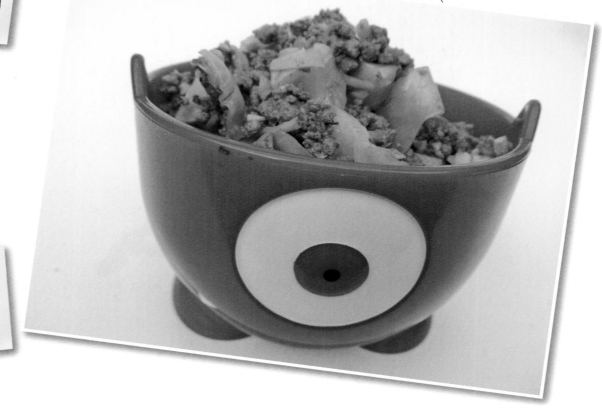

Preheat oven to 325 degrees

Special Tools: Food processor or grater. Dutch oven or roasting pan.

Notes:

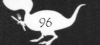
96

Halupki Casserole

Serves 6

Our great grandfather's family is from a country called Hungary. When they get together, they must be REALLY hungry because they bring dozens of stuffed cabbages they call halupkis. The whole family gobbles them up like they're starving, leaving only crumbs behind.

We thought it would be fun to recreate the dish so that we can make our own at home without the rice that's normally included! We made it even easier by using shredded cabbage instead of rolling the meat into cabbage leaves. But if you have time, using cabbage leaves is fun as well!

INGREDIENTS

- ½ head cauliflower
- ¾ lb ground lamb
- ¾ lb ground chuck
- 1 onion, diced
- 3 garlic cloves, minced
- 2 Tbsp olive oil
- ½ head of green cabbage, chopped into ¼-inch ribbons

- 1 (14 oz) can diced tomatoes
- 1 cup tomato sauce
- 1 tsp dried oregano
- 1 tsp paprika
- 2 bay leaves
- salt and pepper to taste
- marinara for serving (optional)

INSTRUCTIONS AND HOW KIDS CAN HELP

1. Cut stems off of cauliflower and use food processor or box grater to make "rice" out of the cauliflower head.
2. In a Dutch oven or roasting pan, brown the meat with the riced cauliflower, onions, garlic, and olive oil—let little hands stir often to incorporate.
3. Add the remaining ingredients and stir to combine.
4. Cover and cook in the oven at 325 degrees for 50 minutes.
5. Serve warm with extra marinara sauce on top.

Main Dishes

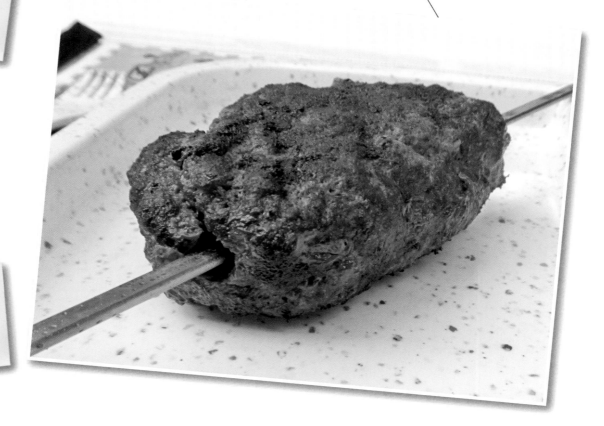

Eat Like a Dinosaur

RAT ON A STICK

Serves 4–6 (ten skewers)

Here is an easy way to make any food fun: put it on a skewer! We like to call this one Rat on a Stick because it reminds us of the movie *Shrek* when he roasted rats over the fire for Fiona.

Although we give directions for cooking these in an oven, they can also be cooked really well over a campfire flame or on your grill. The curry paste adds good flavor for kids and parents alike. Feel free to add more curry paste if you prefer a spicier flavor.

This meal is really quick to prepare, so we often cook it in the morning to pack for lunches. It's an excellent pair with our Coconut Cream Sauce (p. 151) or our Thai Curry Coconut Dip (p. 153).

INGREDIENTS

- ⋄ 2 lb ground red meat (we like 1 lb each lamb and beef)
- ⋄ 2 Tbsp Thai red curry paste (This amount will make the meat sweet, not overly hot)
- ⋄ 1 egg
- ⋄ 2 tsp ground cumin seed
- ⋄ 1 tsp salt
- ⋄ 1 tsp paprika
- ⋄ 10 (6-inch) skewers

INSTRUCTIONS AND HOW KIDS CAN HELP

1. Combine all ingredients in a bowl and mix with big and little hands.
2. Form fat mounds of meat around skewers, a bit less than a quarter pound per skewer.
3. Cook in oven at 350 degrees for 20 minutes, flipping halfway through.

Preheat oven to 325 or grill to medium low

Special Tools: Meat thermometer is helpful

Notes:

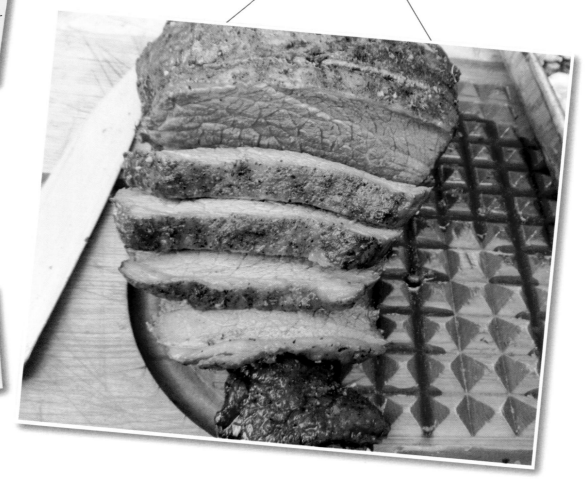

Eat Like a Dinosaur

ROAST BEAST

Serves 6

When we read *How the Grinch Stole Christmas*, one particular part interested us at the end—the part where the Whos eat ROAST BEAST! We wondered what a roast beast might taste like, so we decided to make one ourselves. The biggest beast we could roast was a cow, so this is a beef roast recipe.

We felt more like dinosaurs than Whos when there was a big chunk of meat on our table to dig into!

INGREDIENTS

- ½ tsp garlic powder
- ½ tsp dried basil
- ½ tsp dried rosemary
- 1 Tbsp salt
- ¼ tsp pepper
- 3 lbs beef roast

INSTRUCTIONS AND HOW KIDS CAN HELP

 1. Combine herbs, salt, and pepper in a small bowl and mix with a fork.

2. With hands, rub mixture on all surfaces of beef roast.

3. In 325 degree oven (or over indirect medium-low heat on a grill) roast for 90 minutes until it reaches medium-rare temperature of 135 degrees.

4. Allow to rest uncovered for 10 minutes before cutting.

5. Slice into ½-inch slices and serve.

Some dinosaurs are carnivores and only eat meat. This is probably not a chapter for them. Side dishes are usually full of the vegetables that fuel herbivores like brachiosaurus or stegosaurus. But even if you think you're a junior velociraptor, you can't really survive on hamburgers alone! That's where all these fun ways of making vegetables come in.

Remember, just because you don't like one ingredient doesn't mean all vegetables will be gross to you! Some kids don't like eggplant, but they love zucchini. Some don't love cauliflower, but will scarf down lots of broccoli. You know, dinosaurs had favorite foods too. Sauropods like diplodocus or brachiosaurus ate the leaves on the tops of trees but didn't eat grass. Triceratops and stegosaurus may have eaten grass, but didn't eat eggs. Oviraptors ate eggs, but didn't eat swamp weeds. Parasaurolophus and other duckbill dinosaurs ate that. Find your favorite vegetables and eat those!

It's also important to remember that your taste buds change (did you know your tongue changes its skin just like snakes?). And things you didn't like six months ago may end up being your favorite just a little while later. Our rule is that we always try just one bit of everything on the table so we can see if our taste buds have changed or not. Hopefully your parents will make foods that are your favorite more often than foods that aren't your favorite. If you keep trying new foods, you will learn what's good to you!

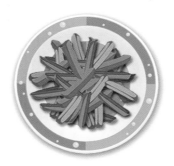

CHAPTER 4
SIDE DISHES

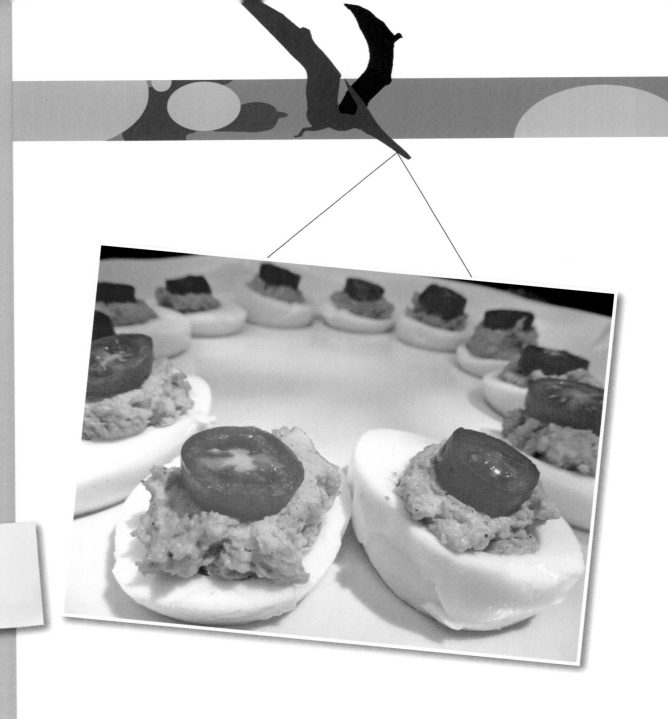

Notes:

Eat Like a Dinosaur

DEVILED BACONY EGGS

Serves 4

Deviled eggs are hard-boiled eggs that have the yellow yolk in the middle taken out, mixed up with yummy stuff, and then stuffed back into the white. Often you'll find deviled eggs at parties sitting out on a buffet. They're so yummy; our boys eat them like candy. Ours may look a little different, but they are delicious!

Usually, they're made with mayonnaise, so rather than use the kind from the store, we used our Bacon Mayonnaise (p. 137) to give them extra flavor. If you want them to taste like eggs and not bacon, use our Mayonnaise (p. 137)—but we recommend giving the Bacon Mayonnaise a shot.

We like to top our deviled eggs with a tomato slice, wrap them in lettuce, and pop them in our mouths. We call it a BLT Popper. How would you eat them?

INGREDIENTS

- 6 eggs
- ¼ C Bacon Mayonnaise (p. 137)
- ½ Tbsp salt
- ½ tsp vinegar
- ¼ tsp paprika
- ¼ tsp dry mustard
- dash of salt and pepper
- optional: 6 sliced grape tomatoes, chives or crumbled bacon

INSTRUCTIONS AND HOW KIDS CAN HELP

1. To make hard-boiled eggs, first put large eggs of similar size in a sauce pan and cover with water plus an extra half inch, a pinch of salt, and a splash of vinegar.
2. Bring to boil uncovered over high heat.
3. Boil for one minute, then remove from heat and cover in hot water for 20 minutes.
4. Place cooked eggs into an ice bath to stop cooking.
5. When cooled, peel eggs out of their shell.
6. Slice eggs in half vertically and remove yolks with a spoon.
7. In small bowl, mash yolks into a paste with a fork or masher.
8. Add remaining ingredients to yolk and mix until combined.
9. Fill egg whites with yolk mixture and top with sliced tomatoes.

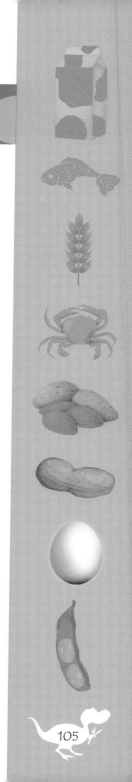

Side Dishes

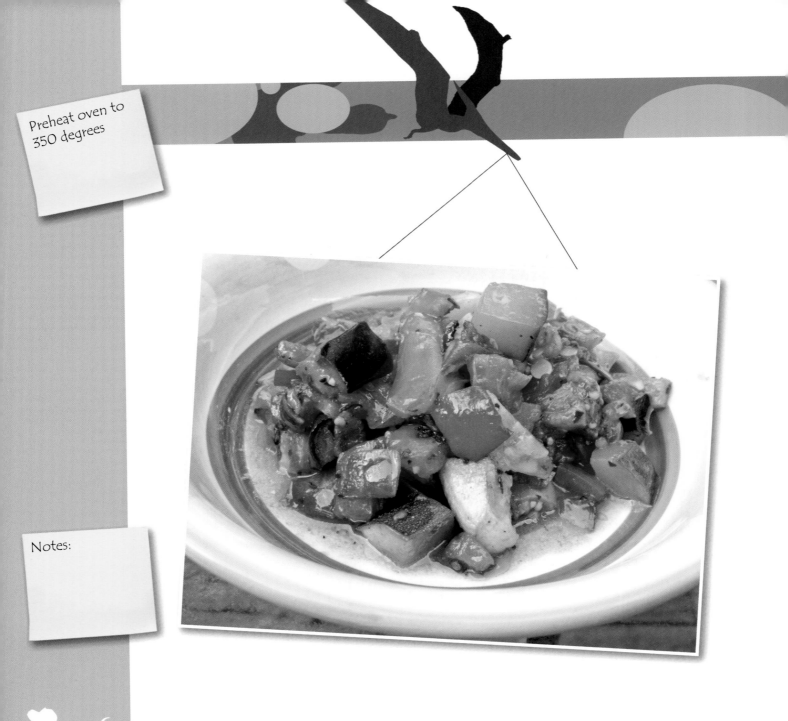

Preheat oven to 350 degrees

Notes:

Eat Like a Dinosaur

RATATOUILLE

Serves 6–8

You know the movie *Ratatouille* about the mouse who cooks? When we watched the movie, we wanted to make ratatouille for ourselves! We were able to find the ingredients all at our local farmers' market on a weekend in July. It was cool to find all the different colors of vegetables. Did you know they have white eggplants? Have you ever seen purple tomatoes? There's even squash that's striped like a tiger! New foods are really exciting and we love to go on a food adventure discovering new stuff— this recipe is the perfect start.

This recipe makes so much ratatouille that we had it for lunch for almost a whole week! Next time we made it, we put it in containers for the freezer, so it's easy to save and have the fresh flavors of summer when it's snowy.

INGREDIENTS

- 2 medium-sized eggplants, diced ½ inch
- 2 bell peppers, diced ½ inch
- 2 large tomatoes, diced ½ inch
- 1 large zucchini, diced ½ inch
- 1 large yellow squash, diced ½ inch
- 1 red onion, peeled
- 1 (14.5 oz) can stewed tomatoes
- 3 Tbsp lard or olive oil, divided

- 2 cloves of garlic, minced
- ¼ cup Bone Stock (p. 133)
- 1 tsp thyme
- ½ tsp rosemary
- ½ tsp sage
- 1 tsp salt
- ½ tsp pepper

INSTRUCTIONS AND HOW KIDS CAN HELP

Pour the canned tomatoes into a large bowl and, with a masher, crush the canned tomatoes into thick liquid. If you don't have a masher, little hands work perfectly too!

2. Using one tablespoon of oil, sauté the onions, garlic, and eggplant until softened, about 8 minutes.

Once the cooked vegetables are finished, add cooked vegetables and the remaining diced vegetables with broth into large bowl and mix.

Add smashed tomatoes, herbs, salt, and pepper and mix until ingredients are evenly distributed.

Evenly spread remaining oil over 9-by-13-inch glass or other baking dish.

Pour mixed vegetables into baking dish.

7. Cook uncovered at 350 degrees for 45 minutes.

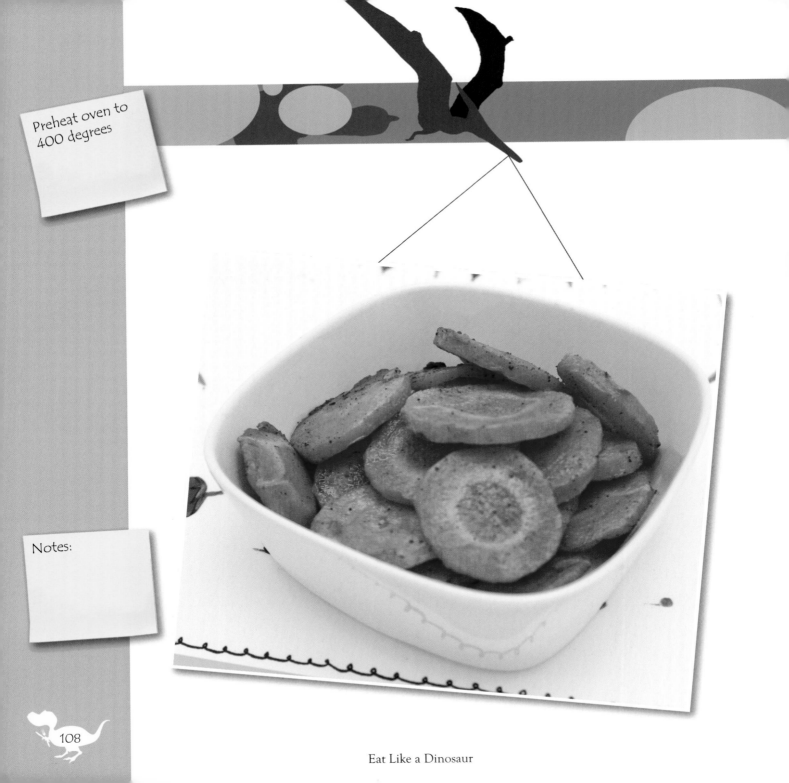

Preheat oven to 400 degrees

Notes:

Eat Like a Dinosaur

Carrot Rounds

Serves 4

If you find really big and thick carrots, this is a perfect way to cut and serve them. If not, this will work with whole baby carrots just as well. Carrots are one of our favorite vegetables; it's a sweet root vegetable that is high in beta-carotene, a super-good-for-you antioxidant that's great for your eyes and skin. We like to serve carrots with nutmeg because it's a perfect complement! Cinnamon is delicious too.

Nutmeg is the seed of a tree that originally only grew on ten tiny islands in the middle of the ocean. It was rare and thought to be a very special seasoning. A few smart people put their heads together and figured out how to share nutmeg all over the world from its tiny home. We're glad it's not rare anymore!

INGREDIENTS

- ◇ 4 large, thick carrots, peeled and sliced into rounds (about 1 pound)
- ◇ 2 Tbsp coconut oil, liquefied
- ◇ 1 tsp salt
- ◇ ½ tsp nutmeg

INSTRUCTIONS AND HOW KIDS CAN HELP

🤚 Toss all ingredients until all carrots are coated.

🤚 Make sure the carrots are in a single layer (we sometimes need to use 2 pans).

3. Roast at 400 degrees for 30 minutes.

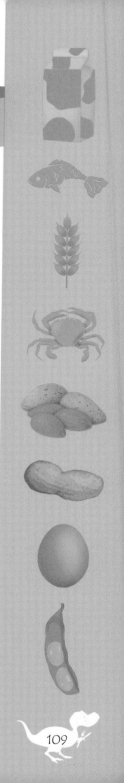

Eat Like a Dinosaur

BUNNY'S SOUP

Serves 8

We checked out a book from a library once about a bunny that loved carrots. The book was pretty silly, because the bunny rabbit was always getting in trouble with a farmer for sneaking into his garden and eating his carrots. At the end was a recipe for carrot soup, which the rabbit shared with his readers. Although that recipe had butter and flour, it gave us the idea to come up with our own version.

This carrot soup is especially delicious because it has a hint of sweetness and a dash of spice. The best part is getting to pour in your own coconut milk before you eat it. Try to see if you can make a fun design when you add it to your bowl; we like to make pretty swirls and heart shapes. It's also fun to make a spider web and have this soup for Halloween!

INGREDIENTS

- 3 Tbsp olive oil or lard
- 16 medium carrots (about 2 pounds) peeled and cut into 2-inch segments
- 1 medium onion (not red), diced
- 3 garlic cloves, minced
- 4 C Bone Stock (p. 133)

- 2 Tbsp yellow curry powder
- 1 tsp cinnamon
- 1 tsp salt
- 1/8 tsp cayenne pepper (optional)
- water to thin (about 1 cup)
- 1 (14 oz) can full-fat coconut milk (optional)

INSTRUCTIONS AND HOW KIDS CAN HELP

1. Heat lard or olive oil in large stock pot over medium heat.
2. Sauté carrots, onion, and garlic for 5 minutes until they begin to soften, letting little hands stir occasionally.
3. Pour in stock and spices; stir.
4. Bring to a boil over high heat and cook 15–20 minutes or until carrots are very soft.
5. Blend soup until smooth, return to heat.
Caution: do not fill blender past halfway to prevent hot spray!
6. Add water and stir until soup is preferred consistency (more or less to your liking).
7. Serve with coconut milk. Stir and mix in coconut milk for a fun activity that adds a rich taste and cuts the heat of the spices.

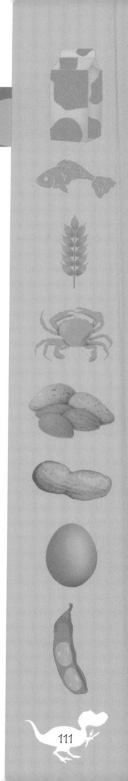

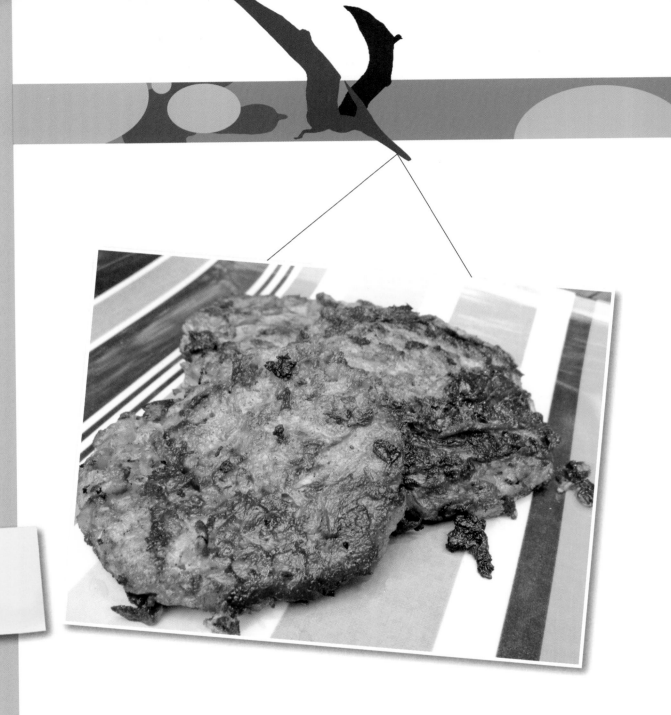

Notes:

Eat Like a Dinosaur

ZUCCHINI LATKES

Serves 4

What are latkes you ask? Well, I know them as little potato pancakes that I like to eat with applesauce. Since we missed them we thought these fun and surprising little green cakes would be a good substitute. They're even better, actually! They're slightly sweet and a delicious addition to your normal eggs in the morning. Add bacon and eggs and you'll have a plate resembling green eggs and ham!

Once these are hot and ready, serve them with a traditional topping—Applesauce (p. 131)! They're also great served as a savory side with chicken for dinner. You could even store them in the fridge when you want an on-the-go snack.

We promise, you will like them in a house, you will like them with a mouse. Perhaps even on a train, but make sure they're allowed on a plane before you pack them in your bag!

INGREDIENTS

- 1 medium zucchini, peeled and grated (about 1½ cups)
- dash of salt
- 1 egg
- 1 Tbsp cinnamon
- 1 Tbsp honey
- 1 tsp vanilla
- 3 Tbsp coconut oil, plus more as needed

INSTRUCTIONS AND HOW KIDS CAN HELP

1. Add zucchini to a mesh strainer, sprinkle with salt and drain for 30 minutes, press out as much liquid as you can or else this will become more of a moist pancake than a crispy patty.

2. Combine strained zucchini, egg, cinnamon, honey and vanilla in a bowl and mix with little hands.

3. Form into patties, about 3 inches diameter and about ½ inch thick.

4. Heat coconut oil in medium frying pan over medium heat.

5. Cook zucchini cakes about 6–8 minutes per side until golden brown.

6. Add more oil to pan between batches to prevent sticking and repeat steps until all latkes are cooked.

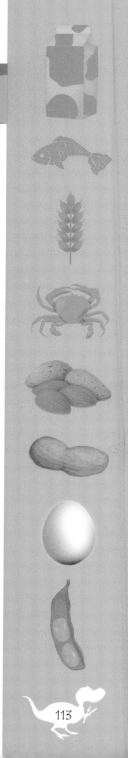

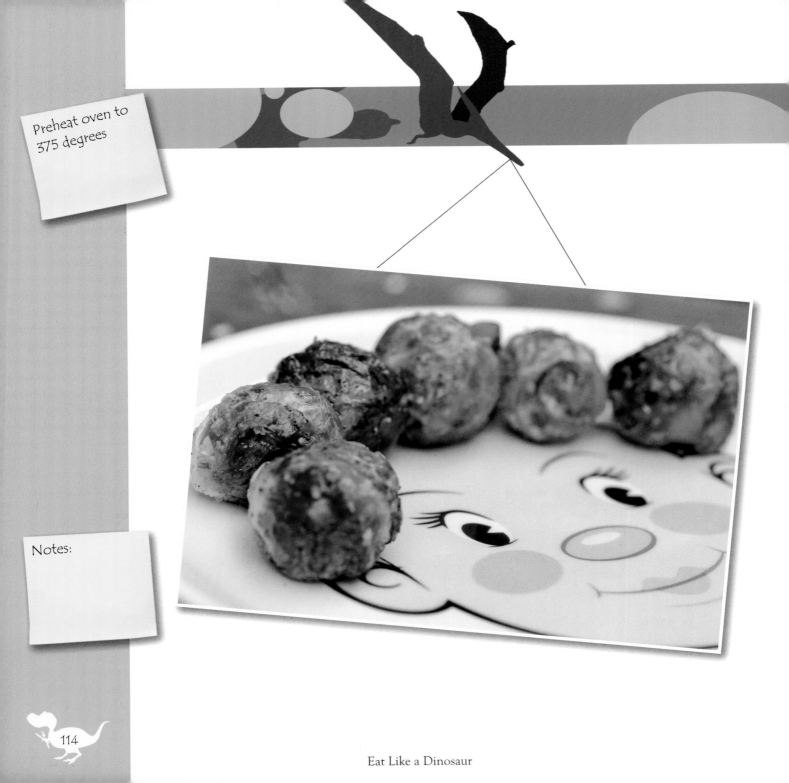

Preheat oven to 375 degrees

Notes:

114

Eat Like a Dinosaur

LITTLE CABBAGE (BRUSSELS SPROUTS)

Serves 6

When we were growing up, Brussels sprouts, or as we like to call them, little cabbages, were famous in movies and TV shows for being yucky to kids. Our boys are lucky they give everything a chance though, because these Brussels sprouts are some of our very favorites!

We love these little baby cabbages just as they are. In the oven they get crispy on the outside and soft on the inside. They're great! Make them this way and we dare you not to love them!

INGREDIENTS

- ⋄ 2 lbs Brussels sprouts
- ⋄ 3 Tbsp melted lard or coconut oil
- ⋄ 1 Tbsp salt
- ⋄ ¼ tsp black pepper

INSTRUCTIONS AND HOW KIDS CAN HELP

 1. Chop ends off of sprouts and remove outer and brown leaves.

2. Toss all ingredients together on large baking sheet.

3. Roast for 30-40 minutes at 410 degrees, or until softened and browned.

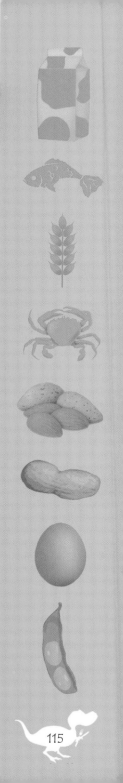

115

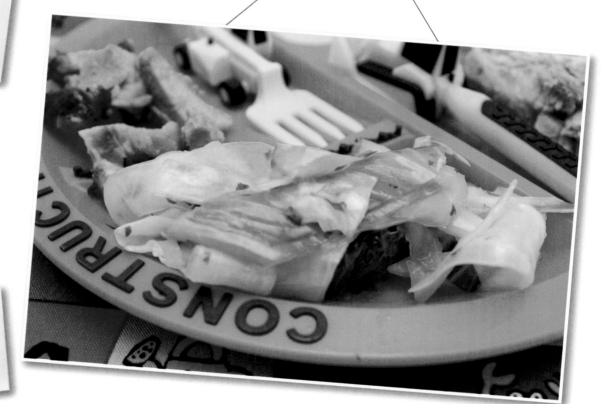

Eat Like a Dinosaur

Chou Vert (Big Cabbage)

Serves 4

One of our favorite restaurants serves food from a country called Vietnam. If you've never tried this kind of food, you should give it a shot! Most Vietnamese restaurants are full of healthy choices for you, and their herbs and spices taste so fresh! Just make sure that what you order doesn't have soy sauce, which often has wheat as a first ingredient.

We wanted to use those Vietnamese flavors at home, so we decided to make this cabbage dish. We wanted to call it something fun, so we called it the French name for cabbage. It's silly and fun to pronounce "shoe verr" when we talk about cabbage for dinner—makes it seem so fancy! We think it makes sense, since French was once spoken in Vietnam.

Ingredients

- 3 Tbsp lard, or duck fat (our favorite)
- 2 cloves garlic, minced
- ½ head of cabbage, sliced into ribbons
- 2 green onions, sliced
- 2 tsp cilantro, chopped fine
- ½ tsp salt

Instructions and How Kids Can Help

1. Melt fat in a frying pan or wok over medium heat.
2. Add garlic and cabbage and toss in pan to coat thoroughly.
3. Continue to cook, stirring often, until cabbage is wilted and slightly browned, 6 minutes.
4. Remove from heat and mix in onion, cilantro and salt.

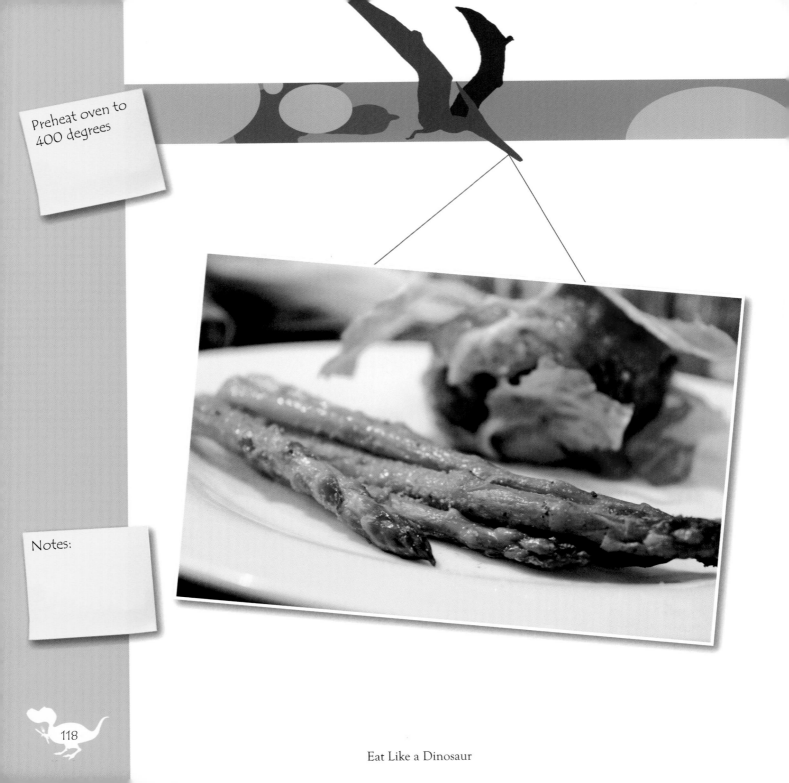

Preheat oven to 400 degrees

Notes:

118

Eat Like a Dinosaur

Nature's Spears (Asparagus)

Serves 4

If you're like our boys, you probably see the world as being full of weapons. Any stick becomes a sword or a gun and any string becomes a whip. Well, it shouldn't be a shock, then, that the first time we had asparagus they were immediately used as spears. That lasted only until our boys put them in their mouths and decided they loved to eat them more than play with them!

Ingredients

- 1 lb asparagus spears
- 3 Tbsp melted lard or olive oil
- 1 tsp salt
- 1 tsp ground cumin
- ¼ tsp pepper

Instructions and How Kids Can Help

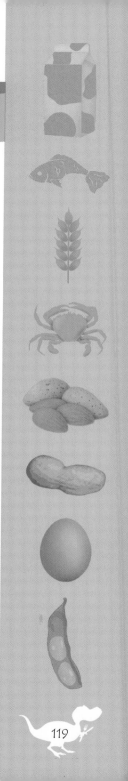

1. Remove the ends of the asparagus by letting your little one find the natural "snap" point when you bend it in half.

2. Toss and coat asparagus with remaining ingredients.

3. Arrange in single layer on baking sheet.

4. Roast asparagus at 400 degrees for 25-30 minutes until asparagus is slightly limp, but still has a bite.

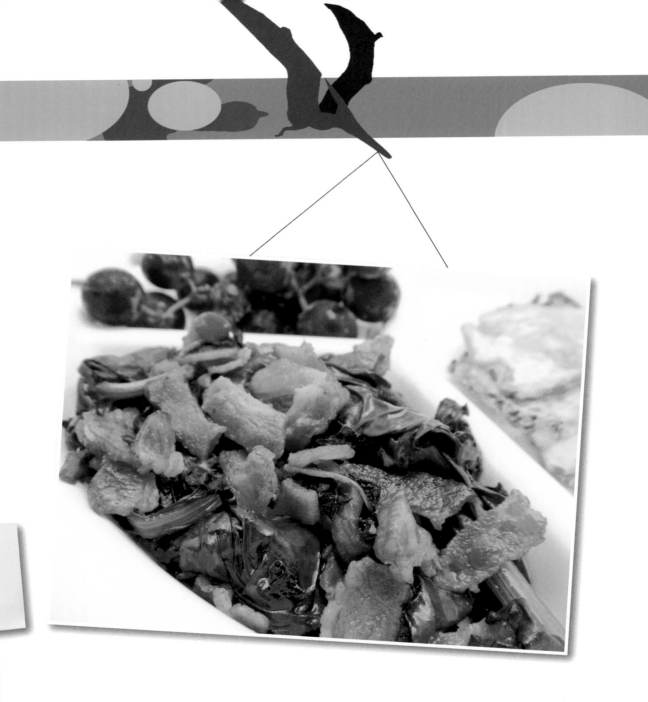

Notes:

120

Eat Like a Dinosaur

GREENS & BACON

Serves 4

Popeye may eat spinach from a can, but we think you'll prefer fresh spinach! You may have had spinach in a salad, but it's really neat to cook spinach because it shrinks in the pan! We also think you'll like spinach better with bacon. Lots of bacon! We eat this with breakfast a lot and it really helps our bodies grow strong because spinach has tons of good vitamins and minerals. And the stable saturated fat from the bacon makes those nutrients easily absorbed by your growing body. Not to mention, bacon makes everything taste better!

INGREDIENTS

- ◇ ½ lb nitrate-free bacon, diced
- ◇ 4 cups spinach (or any fresh green, reuse the tops of your beets and turnips too)
- ◇ ¼ tsp pepper

INSTRUCTIONS AND HOW KIDS CAN HELP

1. Over medium heat, fry bacon until almost crispy.
2. Add spinach and toss quickly to coat with bacon grease.
3. Continue to toss and allow spinach to wilt but not burn, about 3 minutes.
4. Remove from heat and mix in pepper.

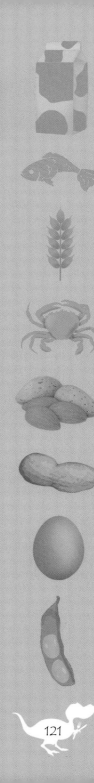

Preheat oven to
350 degrees

Notes:

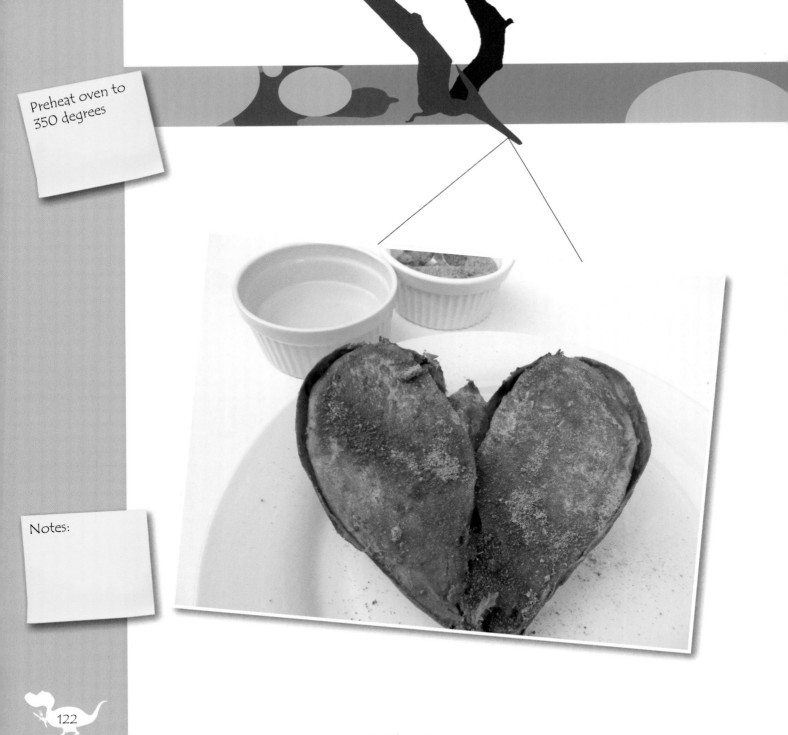

Eat Like a Dinosaur

ROASTED SWEET POTATOES

Serves 4

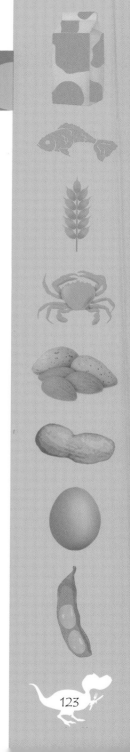

We don't know why sweet potatoes aren't even more loved than white potatoes. They are so much cooler! First, they taste better. Second, they're bright orange! Who doesn't love orange food? We eat orange foods like sweet potatoes, carrots, and pumpkins because they're full of beta-carotene and other vitamins and minerals to help our bodies stay healthy and strong.

We like to use sweet potatoes in a lot of our recipes because they're tasty, but we think you'll especially love them this way because it's like having dessert for dinner!

INGREDIENTS

- ◊ 4 medium sweet potatoes
- ◊ melted coconut oil
- ◊ unrefined granulated sugar

INSTRUCTIONS AND HOW KIDS CAN HELP

 1. Wash potatoes thoroughly.

 2. With fork, poke 8–10 holes into flesh of potato.

3. Wrap potato with single layer of aluminum foil.

4. Roast directly on the oven rack at 350 degrees for 40 minutes, or until tender.

You can also use an outdoor grill, cook over medium indirect heat.

5. Carefully unwrap cooked potato.

 6. Serve with a drizzle of coconut oil and a sprinkle of palm sugar.

123

Side Dishes

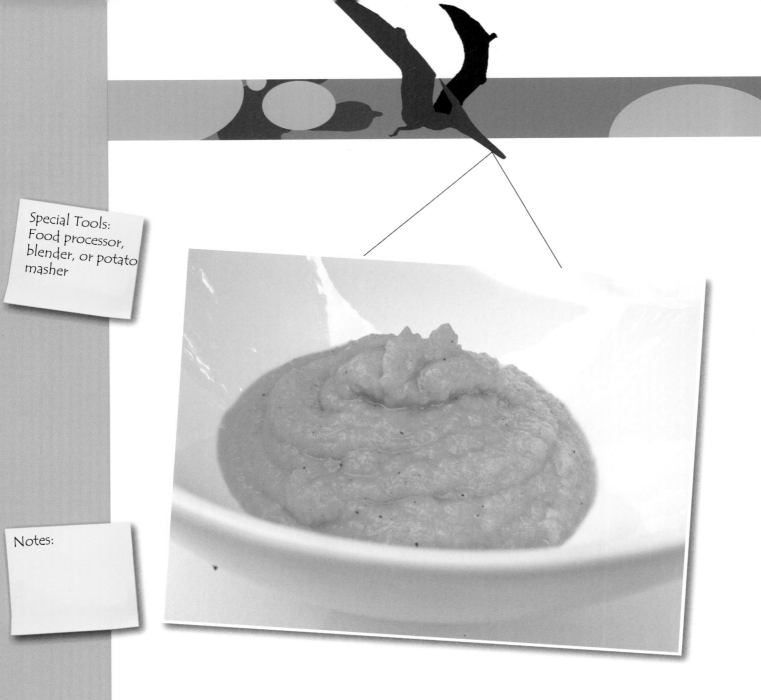

Special Tools:
Food processor,
blender, or potato
masher

Notes:

Eat Like a Dinosaur

Maple Butternut Squash Purée

Serves 4–6

Butternut squash is an interesting vegetable that's shaped like a bell and is light orange on the inside. We get so excited when we start to see this funny-shaped squash arrive in the farmers' market. It's super-easy to grow in your garden, too. Every year we try to grow the largest squash we can.

What's great about butternut squash is that it's slightly sweet and rich without needing to do much to it. We like to roast it and make soup with it too. In this recipe, it gets even better with the addition of maple syrup and nutmeg. Use this purée as a side dish or even as a dip. One of our friends told us they even eat it for dessert!

Ingredients

- ◇ 1 butternut squash, peeled and cut into 1-inch cubes
- ◇ ½ C full-fat canned coconut milk
- ◇ 2 Tbsp melted lard or olive oil
- ◇ 1 Tbsp maple syrup
- ◇ ½ tsp salt
- ◇ ½ tsp nutmeg

Instructions and How Kids Can Help

1. Cook squash in boiling water for 10 minutes until tender.
2. Strain from cooking liquid and transfer squash to food processor.
3. Pulse purée squash or mash until smooth.
4. Add remaining ingredients and pulse until incorporated.

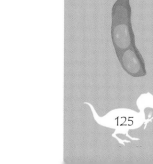

Notes:

126

Eat Like a Dinosaur

Sweet Potato Fries

Serves 4–6

Did you know that French fries are made out of white potatoes? White potatoes aren't particularly nutritious; in fact, their skin can be hard for some people's bodies to use as fuel. So they are not something we often eat. With these fries made out of sweet potatoes, which we think are even tastier because of their sweet flavor, you get the fun of fries with a much healthier approach. The next time you have hamburgers, consider making these.

INGREDIENTS

- ◇ 2 lbs sweet potatoes, peeled
- ◇ ½ C coconut oil
- ◇ 2 tsp salt
- ◇ 2 tsp cinnamon

INSTRUCTIONS AND HOW KIDS CAN HELP

1. Cut sweet potatoes into fry shapes, about ½ inch by ½ inch by 3 inches.

2. Spread sliced potatoes out on large baking sheet and toss with coconut oil, salt, and cinnamon until coated.

3. Spread evenly, ensuring potatoes are not overly crowded, in a single layer on baking sheet.

4. Roast at 400 degrees for 30 minutes, flipping fries halfway through (alternatively, you could fry them in a deep fryer filled with 325 degree coconut oil).

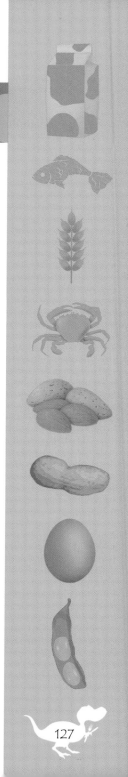

Side Dishes

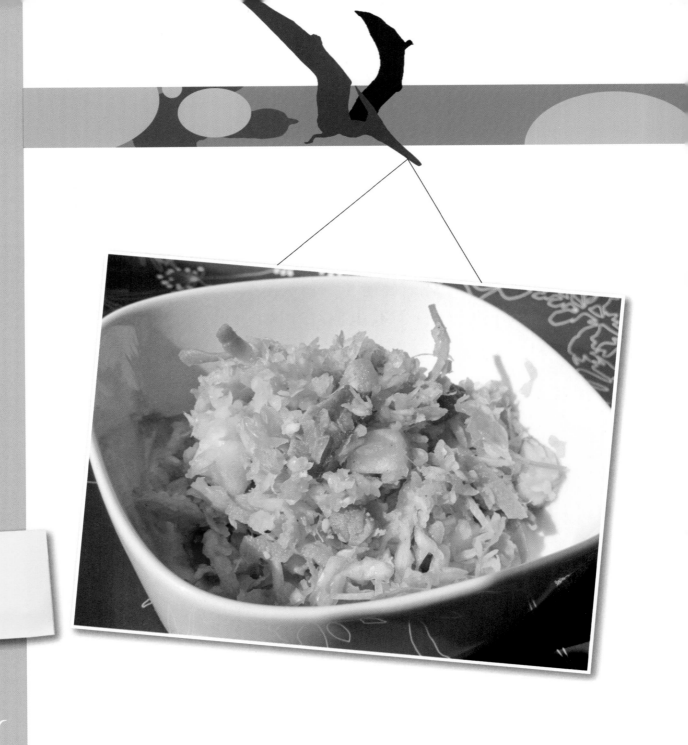

Notes:

Eat Like a Dinosaur

APPLE BACON SLAW

Serves 6

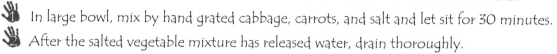

We sometimes call this recipe "Cole's slaw" because it was Cole's idea to add apples and bacon to the coleslaw we used to make. And what an excellent choice it was! This is perfect for eating with barbeque chicken or pork.

Coleslaw is a salad of cabbage and other raw ingredients. Instead of coating ours with thick mayonnaise, we like to flavor it with vinegar for a tangy twist. The apples, bacon, and cumin give it a nice smoky sweet flavor.

INGREDIENTS

- ⋄ ½ head of cabbage, grated
- ⋄ 2 large carrots, grated
- ⋄ 1 Tbsp salt
- ⋄ ⅓ lb bacon (about 5 slices), diced
- ⋄ 1 large apple, diced (skin on will add color and texture)
- ⋄ 1 Tbsp apple cider vinegar
- ⋄ 1 tsp cumin
- ⋄ ¼ tsp black pepper

INSTRUCTIONS AND HOW KIDS CAN HELP

1. In large bowl, mix by hand grated cabbage, carrots, and salt and let sit for 30 minutes.
2. After the salted vegetable mixture has released water, drain thoroughly.
3. Cook bacon over medium heat in frying pan until crispy, about 6 minutes.
4. Add bacon, apple, vinegar, cumin, and pepper to vegetable mixture and toss all ingredients until mixed evenly.
5. Serve warm or cold; will stay fresh for several days refrigerated.

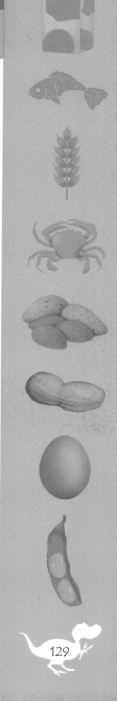

Notes:

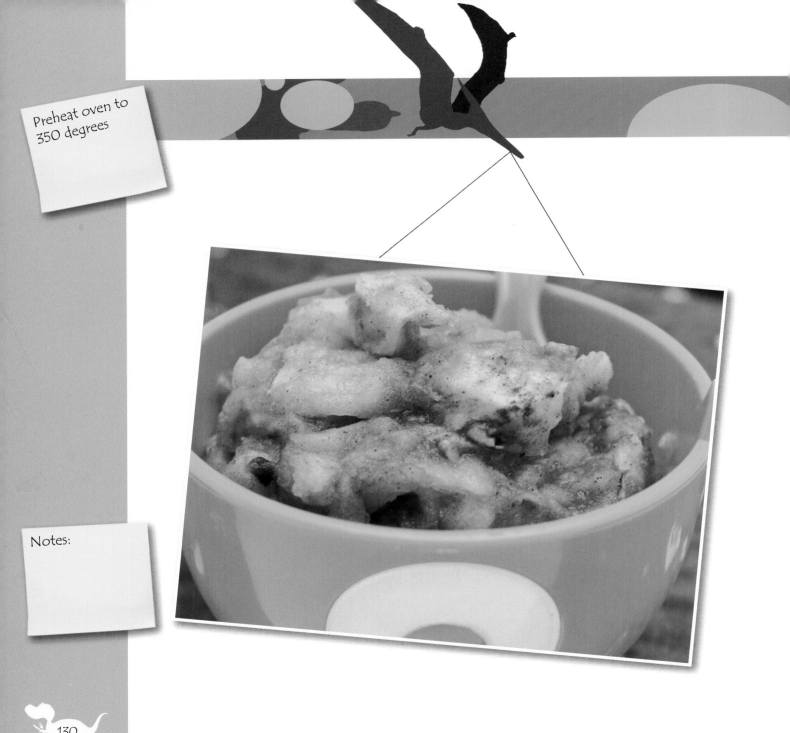

Eat Like a Dinosaur

APPLESAUCE

Makes 4 cups

Have you ever had fresh applesauce made from your own apples? We used to think it was too hard for us to try making it ourselves. But then we gave it a whirl and now we realize it's super-easy and delicious. Now it's almost always in our house, available for snacks at any time or to eat as a side with dinner.

When we get apples we either go to a farm where we pick our own or we go to the farmers' market and buy huge baskets of them. Our farmer gives us a discount for buying a half bushel. That makes lots of Cinnamon Apple Tidbits (p. 167), Apple Rings (p. 165), and this applesauce!

You could also do this in a slow cooker. Just put the apples and cinnamon in for 8 hours on low!

INGREDIENTS

- ◇ 8 apples (baking apples, tart, but not sour—our favorites are York, Fuji, and Honey Crisp)
- ◇ Cinnamon

INSTRUCTIONS AND HOW KIDS CAN HELP

1. Peel all the apples, then section into 8 or more slices (we love our dollar-store apple slicer for this).

2. Place slices in 9-by-13-inch baking dish and sprinkle the top with cinnamon.

3. Bake for 60 minutes at 350 degrees (for a wetter sauce, cover with foil).

4. When apples finish baking, either mash for a chunky sauce or purée for a smooth sauce.

5. Serve warm with pork for dinner or store and serve cold for several weeks—it freezes well too.

Side Dishes

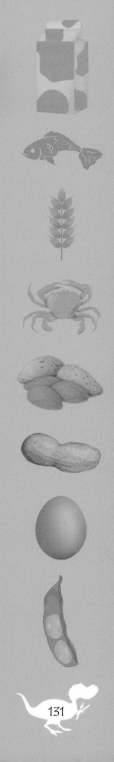

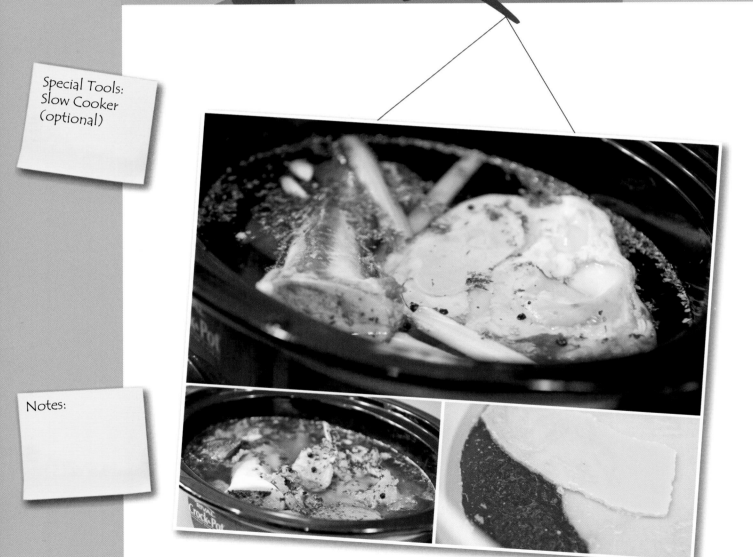

Special Tools:
Slow Cooker
(optional)

Notes:

132

BONE STOCK

Makes 8 cups

Broth is an ingredient often found in recipes. Although you can buy it in the store, making it at home offers a nutrient-dense way to get in calcium, magnesium, and other essential vitamins and minerals. The nutrients are easily and readily absorbed by your body because of the bone marrow's natural healthy fat. With the natural gelatin of the bones, when you put this broth in the fridge you'll get beef Jell-O! Simply heat the broth up and the layer of fat and gelatin will turn into a delicious and flavorful broth.

And if you make it yourself, then you don't have to buy boxes or cans of broth at the store, which often have "natural flavors"—another word for MSG or weird food like cellulose, made from the wood of trees. I don't know about you, but those ingredients make us a little scared and certainly make our boys' bodies go crazy!

We love cooking with bones. What a fun learning experience! Plus this recipe has the extra benefit of making your house smell delicious for hours! After it's done, you can use it in recipes like our Ratatouille (p. 107) and Bunny's Soup (p. 111), or just have a mug full to start your day!

INGREDIENTS

- ◇ 4 lbs beef bones or 1 whole chicken carcass
- ◇ 4 carrots, broken in half
- ◇ 4 celery sticks, broken in half
- ◇ 2 bay leaves
- ◇ 1 large onion, skinned and quartered
- ◇ 1 head of garlic, halved across the cloves
- ◇ 1 Tbsp salt
- ◇ 1 Tbsp whole black peppercorns
- ◇ 1 tsp mustard seeds
- ◇ 8 C water

INSTRUCTIONS AND HOW KIDS CAN HELP

1. Place all ingredients in a stock pot or slow cooker, covering with water.
2. If using pot on stovetop, cook on high until boiling, then cover and reduce heat to low; if using slow cooker, set to low.
3. Simmer chicken stock for 6 hours or 12 hours for beef.
4. After cooking, strain stock to remove remaining vegetable and bone solids.
5. To skim the fat from the broth, place stock uncovered in refrigerator overnight and remove hardened layer the next day—set aside for cooking.
6. Store in sealed containers in refrigerator or freezer.

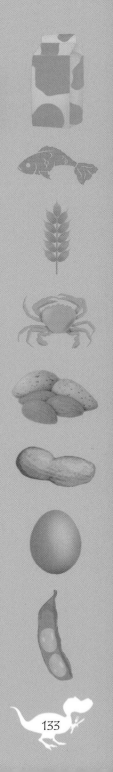

If you're anything like the other children we've met, you probably think that everything is better when it comes with a dip or sauce to pour over it. We agree. In fact, we think you're crazy if you don't like to dip! What's not to love? Adding a dip can turn a carrot into something sweet, spicy, or salty.

Many animals like to dip, too. Did you know that? Raccoons and otters always put their food in the river. Some apes even smear fruit on their vegetables. If you've ever seen monkeys at the zoo, you know how messy they get, right? Maybe dinosaurs did the same thing. No matter what, we think it's a great idea that you should try too.

What's great about the dips and sauces in this section is that they're all made with ingredients to help you grow big and strong, just like the other food in the book. So, go ahead and use our Fool's Gold (p. 81) as a spoon to get as much dip into your roaring mouth and rumbling belly as quickly as you can!

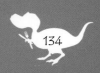

134

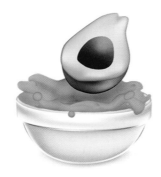

CHAPTER 5
DIPS AND SAUCES

Notes:

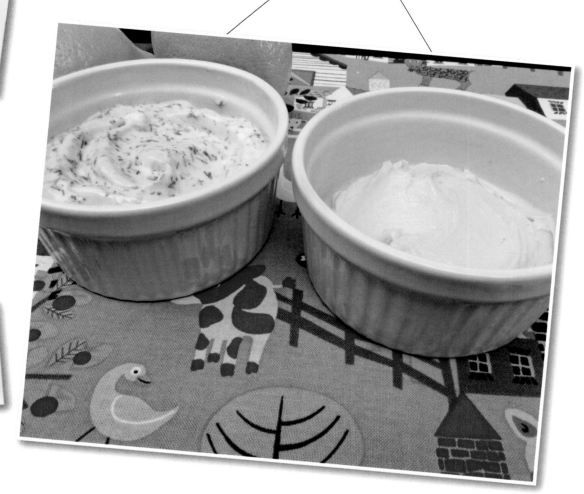

136

MAYONNAISE

Makes a cup of mayonnaise

If you're the type of person that is always whipping out the Miracle Whip or heaping on the Hellmann's, this is for you. Rather than buying sugary mayonnaise made with unhealthy oils, why not make your own? It's pretty easy to do and, once you understand how to do it, it gives you the chance to flavor the mayonnaise any way you'd like!

You can try bacon mayonnaise by replacing the oil with melted bacon grease. If you'd like to add herbs at the end, try lemon zest and dill. It makes a great flavor with fish.

INGREDIENTS

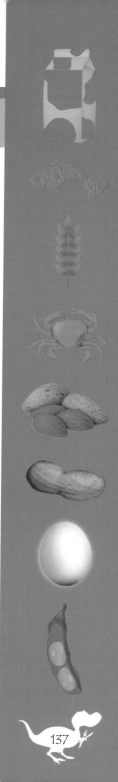

MAYONNAISE

- 2 egg yolks
- 2 tsp lemon juice
- 1 tsp vinegar
- ½ tsp Dijon mustard
- pinch of salt
- ¼ C olive oil
- ½ C macadamia oil (If you don't have macadamia oil, then use avocado oil, coconut oil (liquefied), or entirely olive oil)

BACONNAISE

- 2 egg yolks
- 2 tsp vinegar
- ½ tsp Dijon mustard
- ¾ C bacon fat (liquefied)

LEMON DILL MAYOLI

- 2 egg yolks
- 2 tsp lemon juice
- 1 tsp vinegar
- ½ tsp Dijon mustard
- ¾ C olive oil
- zest of 1 lemon
- 2 tsp dill

INSTRUCTIONS AND HOW KIDS CAN HELP

1. Whisk (we recommend electric, but you can do it by hand too) together the egg yolks, lemon juice, vinegar, mustard, and salt until well combined.
2. Slowly, slowly, slowly (like a sloth) drip in the oil while whisking hard, about 5 minutes.
3. Continue to whisk until the mayonnaise forms to your preferred consistency. This may take up to another five minutes if whisking by hand.

Dips and Sauces

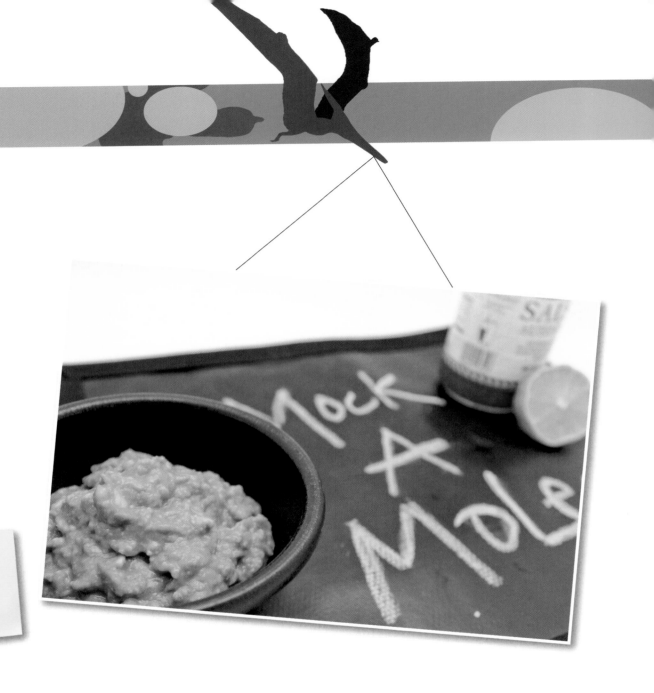

Notes:

138

Mock-a-Mole

Makes 2 cups

Sometimes we put forth the effort to make a real guacamole, but considering how often it's requested in our house, we usually use this simple recipe to create a quick dip our kids use for just about everything! It's nice to make this way because you don't need fresh, ripe tomatoes on hand.

Try putting this dip on your hamburgers and fried eggs or use it for dipping vegetables like cauliflower, carrots, and sweet peppers.

INGREDIENTS

- ⋄ 2 avocados, pit and skin removed
- ⋄ ¼ C red salsa
- ⋄ Juice of ½ lime
- ⋄ ¼ tsp salt

INSTRUCTIONS AND HOW KIDS CAN HELP

1. Mash avocado until most of the chunks are broken up.
2. Mix in salsa, lime juice, and salt until thoroughly combined.

Special Tools:
Food processor
or blender

Notes:

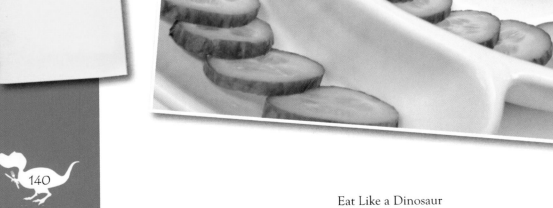

Eat Like a Dinosaur

Black Olive Tapenade

Makes 1 cup

Our boys love black olives. They like them sliced into dishes and salads, they like them plain for putting on their finger tips and popping off with their mouths, and they love them in this tapenade, an olive-based dip.

Since olives are a wonderfully affordable source of lots of good vitamins and minerals, as well as healthy fats, we make olives available as often as the boys ask for them. Try this dip with cucumber, carrots, or even rolled up in pepperoni slices—yum!

INGREDIENTS

- ◇ 1 (6 oz) can black olives, strained and rinsed
- ◇ 1 C raw walnuts
- ◇ 1 garlic clove
- ◇ ½ tsp salt
- ◇ 1 Tbsp vinegar
- ◇ ⅓ C olive oil

INSTRUCTIONS AND HOW KIDS CAN HELP

1. In food processor or blender, purée olives and walnuts for one minute on high.
2. Add garlic, salt, and vinegar and pulse a few times.
3. With processor on high, pour in oil in thin stream until a thick paste forms (scrape the sides and blend again until smooth).
4. Serve at room temperature or cold; store in the refrigerator for at least a week.

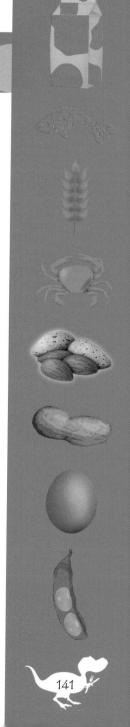

Dips and Sauces

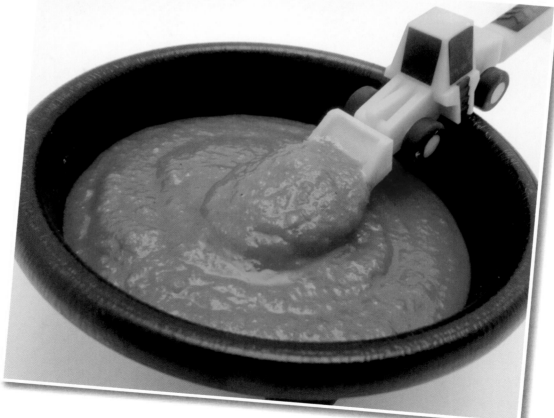

Notes:

142

Ten Tomato Ketchup

Makes 4 cups, enough to refill a squeeze bottle

We love ketchup, and we're willing to bet that you do too. But, do you know what the number two ingredient in most brands of ketchup is? SUGAR! Turns out, the companies that make ketchup don't remove the seeds, since it is extra work. The seeds are yucky and bitter, which is why they need to use sugar to make it taste sweet.

Even Fini didn't think that was good idea, so he agreed to help us remove the seeds of a box of tomatoes. We got them on sale from our farmers' market, and they were super ripe so that we could make our own ketchup without sugar or food color or wheat.

When Cole tasted it for the first time he said, "Mmm, it tastes like tomatoes!" We think that's just how it should taste . . . a little different but worth the time it takes to make it. It's so fresh and healthy you really can put it on just about anything!

INGREDIENTS

- 10 ripe red tomatoes, about 8 cups—the sweeter the variety the better (ask your farmer!)
- 1 medium onion (not red), diced
- 3 cloves garlic, minced
- 2 Tbsp lard
- 2 tsp paprika

- ½ tsp mustard powder
- ¼ tsp ground cloves
- 1 tsp salt
- ¼ tsp pepper
- ¼ C apple cider vinegar
- 2 Tbsp coconut aminos

INSTRUCTIONS AND HOW KIDS CAN HELP

1. Score a shallow X on the bottom of each tomato with a paring knife.
2. Place tomatoes in boiling water for 30 seconds.
3. Remove from boiling water and place into ice bath.
4. Peel off tomato skin, slice in half and remove seeds
5. In large pot over medium heat, sauté onions, garlic, and tomatoes in lard for 8 minutes or until onions start to turn translucent.
6. Add spices, salt, and pepper and simmer for 15 minutes.
7. Blend tomato mixture until smooth, then add back to the pot with onions.
8. Add vinegar and aminos and simmer on medium low for 30 minutes.
9. Add to jar or squeeze bottle and store in refrigerator.

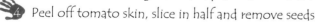

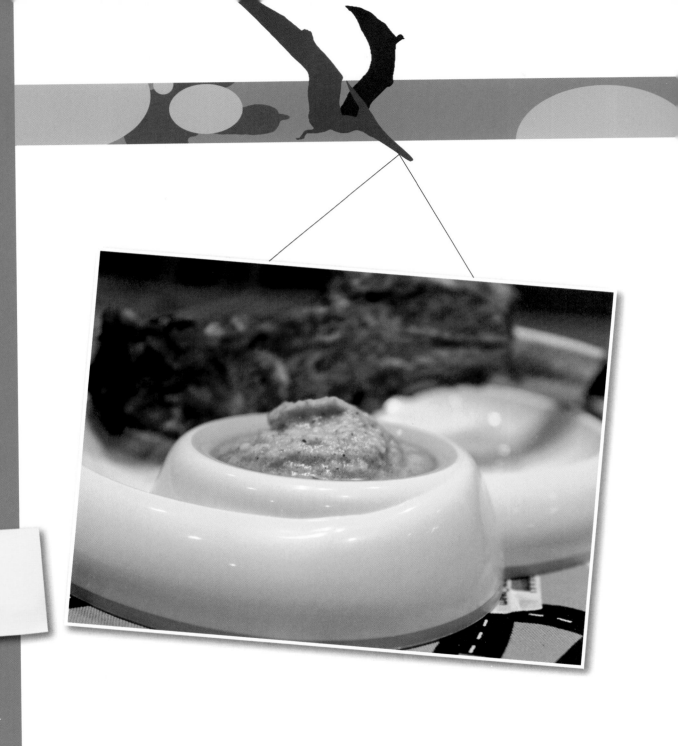

Eat Like a Dinosaur

Texas Barbecue Sauce

Makes 4 cups

Barbecued meat is always better with barbecue sauce. This is our favorite—a sweet version that tastes great on almost any meat. You may not know this, but different states have different barbecue sauces. While this one is like the sauces they make in Texas with ketchup and chili powder, sometimes we will make a Carolina sauce with vinegar or a Kansas City sauce with molasses. This one, however, is our favorite. We especially like it with grilled chicken, beef, and pork, like our Shakey Pork Backbone on p. 53.

Some people say that making a good BBQ sauce is something that takes a lifetime to master, but with this sauce you'll be able to make it in just a short time. It's finger-lickin' good, so make sure to get a dipping bowl for the next time your family barbecues meat!

INGREDIENTS

- ½ C onion, diced
- ½ C celery, diced
- 3 garlic cloves, minced
- ¼ C lard
- 1 C Ketchup (p. 143) or a brand without sweetener
- ½ C cider vinegar
- 1 C Bone Stock (p. 133) or water
- ½ C coconut aminos
- 1 tsp ground pepper
- 1 Tbsp chili powder

INSTRUCTIONS AND HOW KIDS CAN HELP

1. Sauté onion, garlic, and celery in lard over medium heat; cook until softened (about 15 minutes).
2. Add ketchup, vinegar, broth or water, aminos, and pepper.
3. Simmer on low heat, uncovered, for 20 minutes.
4. Stir in chili powder and cook 5 additional minutes.
5. Blend sauce until smooth (optional).
6. Let sit at room temperature for an hour for flavors to develop; store refrigerated for up to several months.

Special Tools:
Blender or food
processor

Notes:

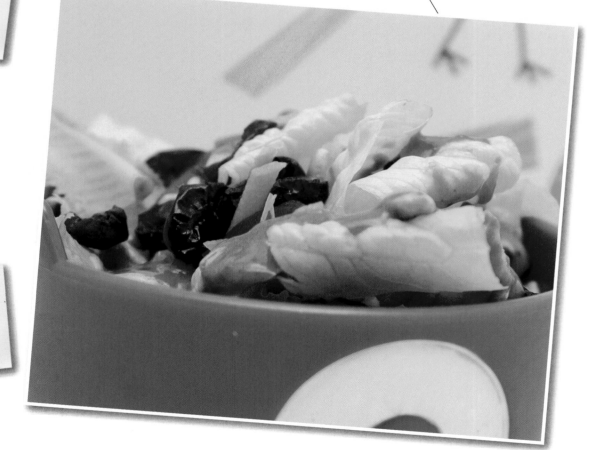

Eat Like a Dinosaur

Raspberry Dressing

Makes 1½ cups of dressing

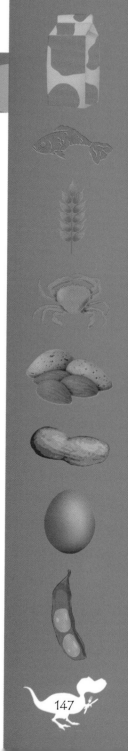

If you use your imagination to think about interesting ingredients and unusual dressings, salads can be fun and delicious. Most days, we like our salads to have fruit, and this dressing is a perfect compliment. It's made with raspberries and naturally results in a cool bubble-gum pink color. How fun is that?!

Ingredients

- 1 C frozen raspberries
- ½ cup water
- 1 Tbsp lemon juice
- 1 Tbsp vinegar
- 1 tsp brown or Dijon mustard
- ¼ tsp pepper
- ¼ C olive oil

Instructions and How Kids Can Help

1. In medium saucepan, simmer raspberries and water over medium heat for about 10 minutes until thickened—letting little hands stir occasionally.
2. Purée until smooth.
3. If you like a smooth dressing, strain with mesh strainer (we skip this step and enjoy the texture of the seeds), then return to blender.
4. Add lemon juice, vinegar, mustard, and pepper and pulse to combine.
5. Slowly add olive oil to purée until completely emulsified.
6. Transfer to an airtight container and keep up to several weeks; keep chilled up to several months.

Special Tools:
Food processor
or blender

Notes:

Eat Like a Dinosaur

SOUTHWESTERN PINEAPPLE SAUCE

Makes about 2 cups of sauce

The most exciting part of this dip is the part where you get to set a pepper on fire! We're not even kidding: to roast the pepper, we use our stovetop burner and roast it like a marshmallow. If you're not able to do that, it can also be done in your oven on the hottest setting. But it's a lot of fun to watch the pepper catch on fire.

When the pepper is nice and roasted, you peel off the burned skin to reveal a smoky and slightly sweet southwestern-flavored pepper perfect for pairing with pineapple! We love this as a dip for carrots, cauliflower, and our Fool's Gold Chicken Nuggets (p. 81). We bet you'll like to put it on fish, veggies, or just about anything!

INGREDIENTS

- 3 medium poblano peppers, roasted
- 1 (20 oz) can pineapple chunks or one whole pineapple
- 2 Tbsp olive oil
- 2 garlic cloves, minced
- 1 Tbsp cider vinegar
- ¼ tsp salt

INSTRUCTIONS AND HOW KIDS CAN HELP

1. Roast peppers, either over an open flame or under the broiler (turning every few minutes) until blackened on all sides.
2. Cover hot peppers (airtight) and let sit for 15 or more minutes; once steamed, the skin of the peppers should peel easily.
3. Peel the skin off of the peppers; run under water if the scorched skin does not peel easily.
4. Purée the peeled peppers and pineapple together (include juice).
5. Over medium heat, heat oil and garlic in a medium saucepan.
6. Cook garlic until just starting to brown, about 4 minutes.
7. Add purée, vinegar, and salt and stir.
8. Simmer for about 20 minutes until a thick sauce is formed; have little hands stir occasionally.
9. Serve cold, store chilled for up to several weeks.

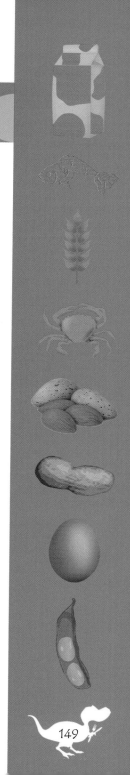

149

Dips and Sauces

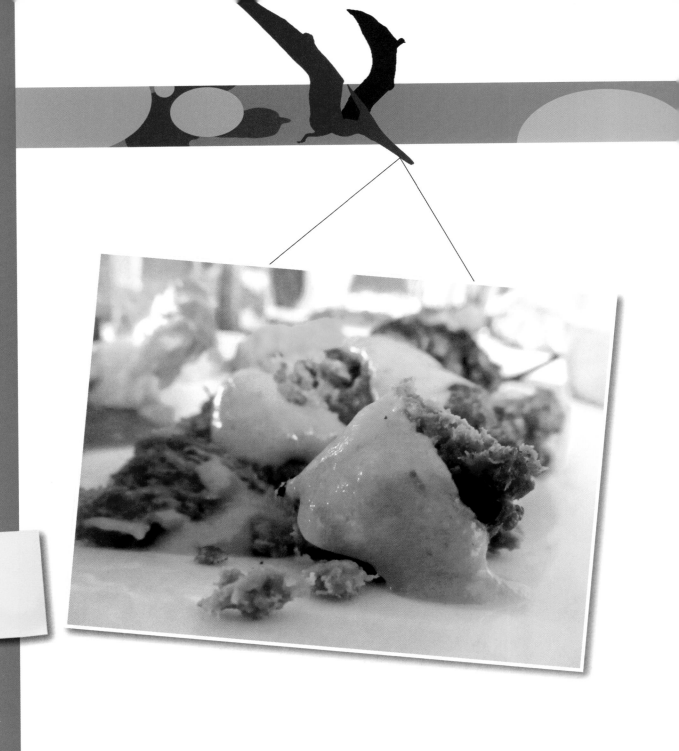

Notes:

150

SAVORY COCONUT CREAM SAUCE

Makes ½ cup

Deep in the jungles of the elephant head–shaped country of Thailand there is a secret. For centuries the culinary geniuses who invented Thai cuisine have magicked together the spicy curries of India with the tropical flavors of the Pacific and a dash of Chinese cookery. The end result is food that combines rich spiciness with tropical playfulness. In honor of that tradition, we bring you a sauce that brings it all together. If all that doesn't make any sense, just know that the people who eat this food also ride elephants—so they must be smarty pants who know what they're doing! Try it on our Rat on a Stick (p. 99) or even with Fool's Gold (p. 81)!

INGREDIENTS

- ⅓ C coconut cream concentrate (alternatively, scoop the cream off the top of a can of full-fat coconut milk)
- 2 Tbsp Thai roasted red chili paste
- 2 tsp cumin
- 1 tsp salt
- 3 Tbsp water to thin

INSTRUCTIONS AND HOW KIDS CAN HELP

1. Combine ingredients in sauce pan over medium heat, stirring constantly.
2. When a paste forms, let little hands add water slowly.
3. Once the sauce coats the back of a spoon, remove from the heat.
4. Sever warm, store chilled for up to several months.

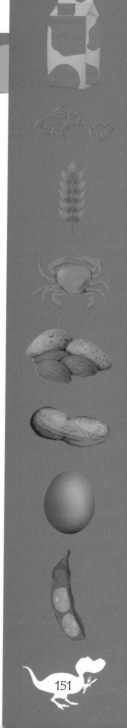

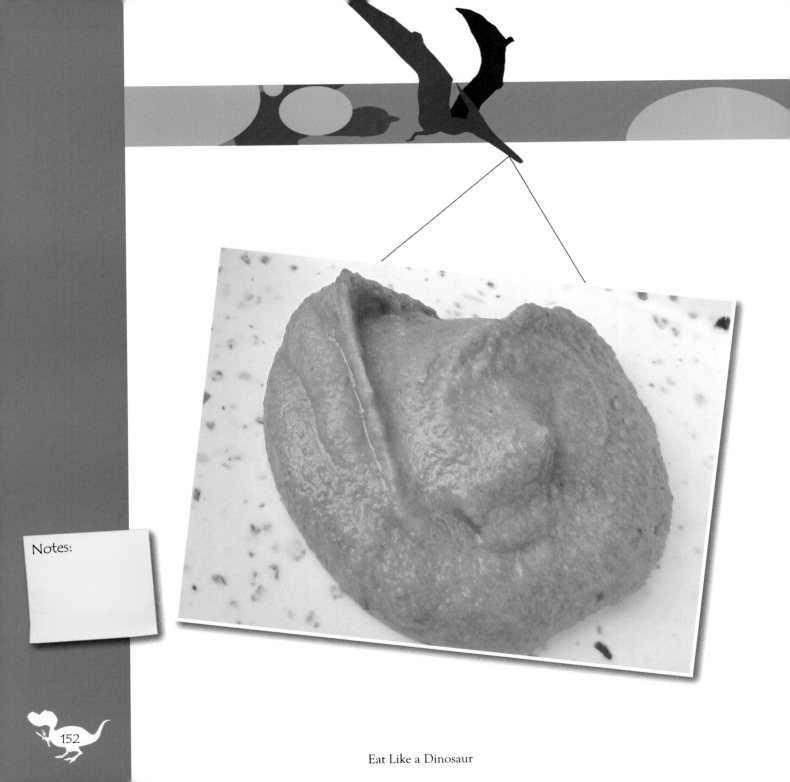

Notes:

Eat Like a Dinosaur

THAI CURRY COCONUT DIP

Makes ½ cup

Go to any party and you'll usually find a veggie plate with carrots, celery, and broccoli, with a tub of ranch dressing in the middle. Instead of that dip, give this fun orange-colored one a try. You'll find an interesting and exotic flavor that will get you excited to dip all the veggies you can!

INGREDIENTS

- ⅓ C coconut cream concentrate (alternatively, scoop the cream off the top of a can of full-fat coconut milk)
- 2 Tbsp Thai red curry paste
- 1 tsp salt
- 1 tsp ground coriander
- 1 tsp lime zest
- 1 Tbsp water to thin

INSTRUCTIONS AND HOW KIDS CAN HELP

1. Combine ingredients in sauce pan over medium heat, stirring constantly.
2. When a paste forms, let little hands add water slowly until the sauce coats the back of a spoon.
3. Turn heat down to simmer for 5-10 minutes until sauce thickens into a dip.
4. Server cold, store chilled for up to several months.

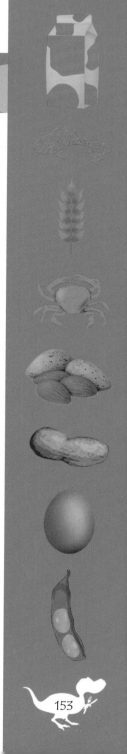

I bet when you've had a long day of school you love running into the kitchen and looking for something to eat. Or maybe if you've been running errands all day in the car, you realize it's been too long since lunch. It's normal and important to refuel, relax, and recharge!

Many dinosaurs were grazers. That means that they just ate all day, munching on whatever food they could find. Some people are like that, too. Cole, for example, always says he's hungry! So, we started making our own snacks for our hatchlings to graze on. Homemade snacks can be delicious and fun to make, but they're especially great to always have around!

What's not to love about making your own healthy cookies, smoothies, or fruit rollups as a snack? Check out our Make Your Own Trail Mix and Make Your Own Fruit & Nut Bars in the Projects chapter for even more ideas. We love these snacks much better than anything we can find in a box; we hope you do too. You can make them, test them, and eat them all with your own claws. We mean hands!

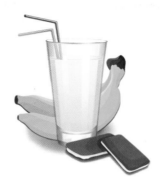

CHAPTER 6
SNACKS

155

Preheat oven to 170 degrees

Special Tools:
Dehydrator
(optional but
recommended)

Notes:

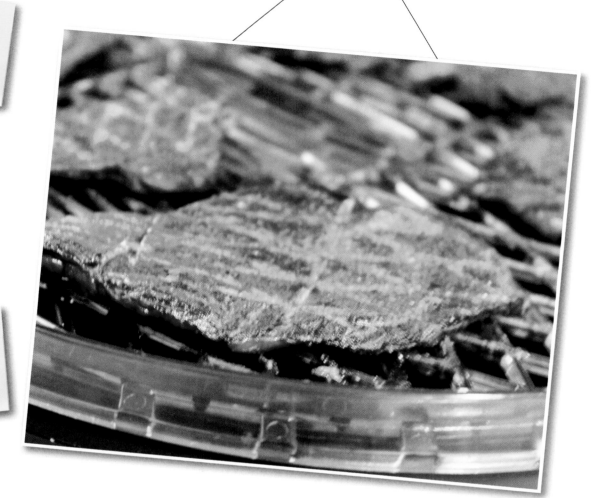

Eat Like a Dinosaur

TERIYAKI BEEF JERKY

Makes about 1½ lbs of jerky

We love beef jerky and, ever since we purchased our favorite kitchen gadget, a dehydrator, we make it all the time. Jerky is a perfect on-the-go snack that is full of protein and has great flavor. It comes in handy when errand running, lasts longer than expected, and helps us avoid scary fast-food options.

INGREDIENTS

- 3 lbs beef (flank steak, London broil, or beef heart)
- ¾ C coconut aminos or wheat-free tamari
- 3 cloves garlic, minced
- 1 Tbsp salt
- 2 tsp cumin
- 1 tsp cinnamon
- ½ tsp pepper

INSTRUCTIONS AND HOW KIDS CAN HELP

1. Carefully slice beef into ¼-inch-thick slices about 2 inches by 3 inches with a knife or mandolin.

2. Whisk remaining ingredients together in a bowl big enough to marinate meat.

3. Microwave for 30 seconds or warm on the stovetop to activate spices.

4. Place meat in marinade and refrigerate for 8 hours or overnight.

5. Dehydrate on medium-high for 4–8 hours or cook at 170 degrees in oven for 12 hours until meat is dry and rubbery (time will vary depending on humidity and the fat content of the meat).

6. Remove jerky and cool in an open container to allow drying to continue. Once cooled, seal container and store in refrigerator or freezer. Jerky can be kept at room temperature, but should be stored long term in cooler temperatures, as there are no preservatives or chemicals to prevent molding.

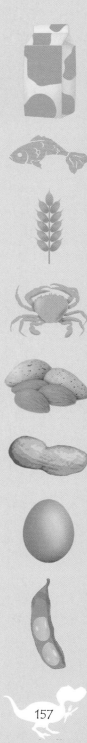

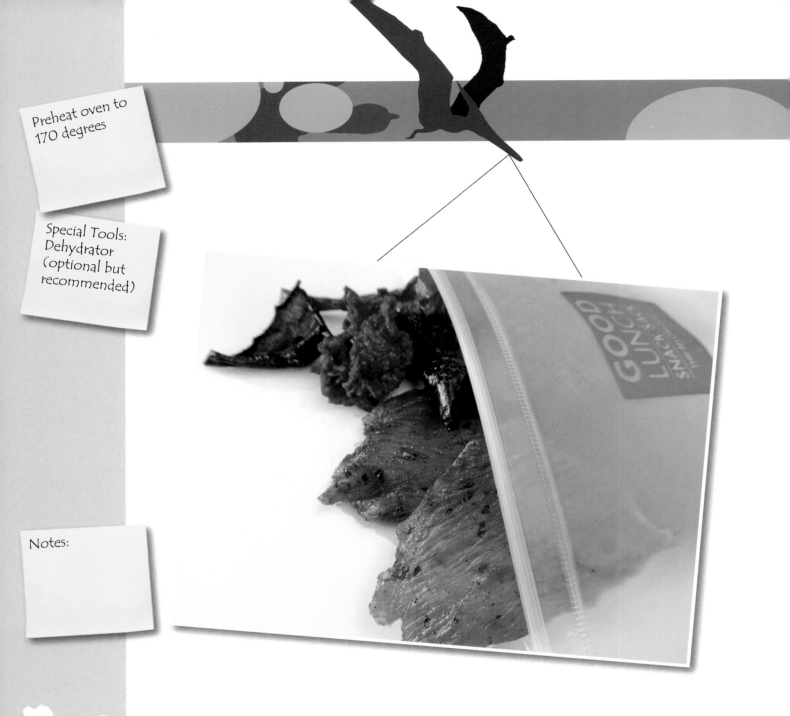

Preheat oven to
170 degrees

Special Tools:
Dehydrator
(optional but
recommended)

Notes:

Eat Like a Dinosaur

TACOS TO GO (CHICKEN JERKY)

Makes about 1 pound of jerky

When you don't eat tortillas, you have to get pretty inventive with how you choose to eat tacos. Since we love beef jerky so much, we decided it'd be fun to have a version for tacos on the go. The dehydrator makes the tomatoes sweet, just like the sundried tomatoes you can buy in the store. And the fun flavors work really well with a different kind of meat—chicken jerky!

INGREDIENTS

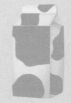

◇	4 chicken thighs	◇	2 tsp chili powder
◇	2 bell peppers	◇	1 tsp salt
◇	2 poblano peppers	◇	1 tsp cumin
◇	2 tomatoes	◇	1 tsp lime juice
◇	¼ C water	◇	1 tsp cilantro, chopped finely
◇	1 Tbsp olive oil	◇	¼ tsp pepper

INSTRUCTIONS AND HOW KIDS CAN HELP

1. Debone and slice chicken into ⅛-inch-thick slices.

2. Slice peppers in to ¼-inch-wide slices.

3. Remove tomato core and slice into ¼-inch-thick slices.

4. Mix remaining ingredients in a bowl with a fork.

5. Microwave marinade for 30 seconds or warm on the stovetop to activate spices.

6. Mix chicken, tomatoes, and peppers with marinade and refrigerate for at least 6 hours.

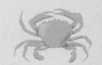

7. Dehydrate meat and vegetable mixture for 4–8 hours at medium-high or bake on baking sheet for 12 hours at 170 degrees (time will vary depending on humidity and the fat content of the meat).

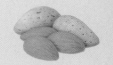

8. Remove jerky and cool in an open container to allow drying to continue. Once cooled, seal container and store in refrigerator or freezer. Jerky can be kept at room temperature, but should be stored long term in cooler temperatures, as there are no preservatives or chemicals to prevent molding.

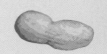

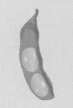

Snacks

Preheat oven to 170 degrees

Special Tools: Dehydrator (optional but recommended)

Notes:

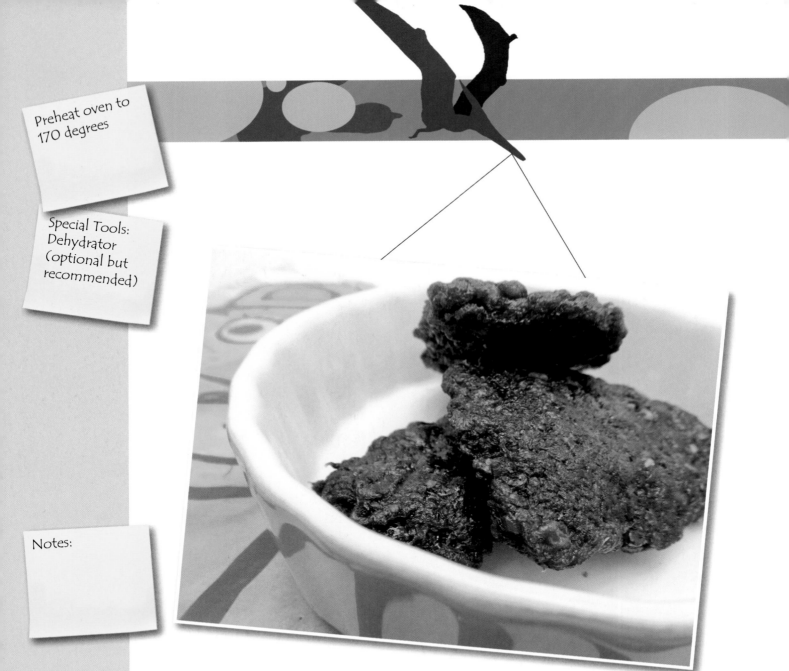

Eat Like a Dinosaur

Honey Barbecue Ground Jerky

Makes about ¾ pound of jerky

Whenever we used to eat fast food, we'd get honey barbeque sauce to dip our meat. It was sweet and tangy—perfect! With this recipe you get to enjoy the flavor of dipping meat without the mess. This slightly sweet, slightly spicy jerky is a terrific snack to take on the go or with a picnic.

To make this recipe a bit different and super easy to make, we chose to use ground meat instead of sliced steak. If you decide to use standard beef slices, you can still use the same delicious marinade!

INGREDIENTS

- ❖ 1 lb very lean ground meat
- ❖ 3 Tbsp honey
- ❖ 1 Tbsp olive oil*
- ❖ 1 Tbsp coconut aminos
- ❖ 1 Tbsp tomato paste

- ❖ 1 Tbsp chili powder
- ❖ 2 tsp salt
- ❖ ½ tsp black pepper
- ❖ note: If you use meat that has natural fat, oil is not necessary

INSTRUCTIONS AND HOW KIDS CAN HELP

1. Mix all ingredients by hand in a bowl until evenly distributed.
2. Allow flavors to develop in refrigerator for at least 6 hours or overnight.
3. Pack tightly into three-by-two-inch patties (meat will shrink), the flatter the better.
4. Dehydrate over medium-high for 4–8 hours or bake in oven at 160 degrees for at least 12 hours (time will vary depending on humidity and the fat content of the meat).
5. Remove jerky and cool in an open container to allow drying to continue. Once cooled, seal container and store in refrigerator or freezer. Jerky can be kept at room temperature but should be stored long term in a refrigerator, as there are no preservatives or chemicals to prevent molding.

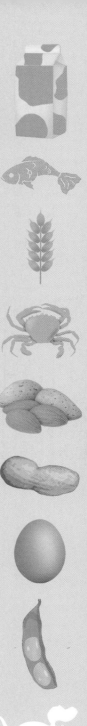

Preheat oven to 400 degrees

Notes:

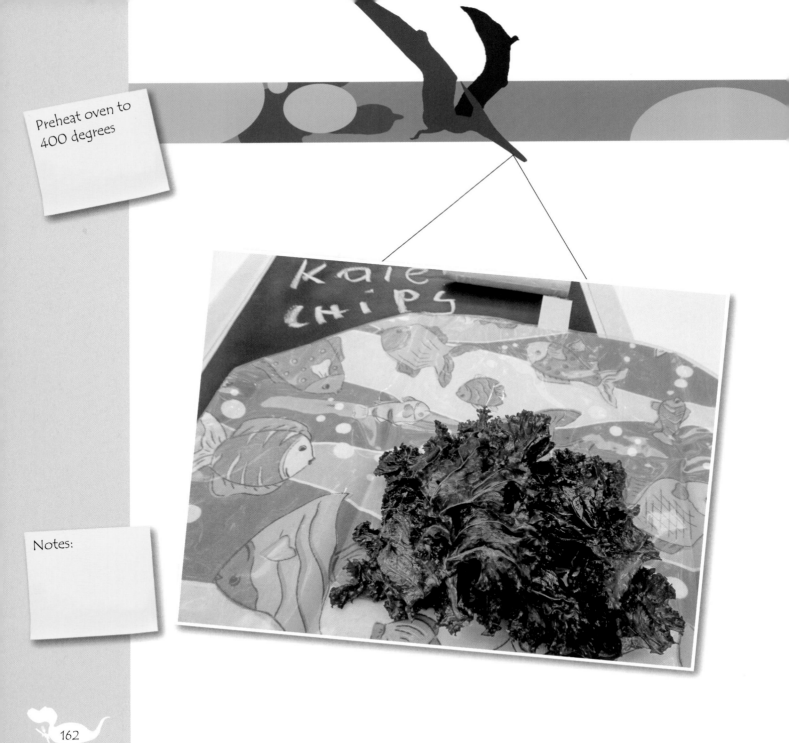

Eat Like a Dinosaur

KALE CHIPS

Makes 3 cups of kale chips

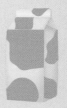

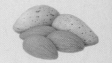
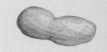

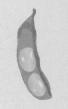

Kale is a "super food" that has dark green, crinkly edges that remind us of ribbons. It's really delicious, especially if you roast it in the oven like this. It turns into crispy chips! When we made this, Cole said, "We made our own seaweed!" because it looked like the dried seaweed he eats in his lunch, but we think it smells and tastes even better.

After you roast it, much of it will get dark, like purple-black dark. That's okay! It's not burnt! It's just extra crunchy!

INGREDIENTS

- ⬥ 1 bunch of kale, about 1 lb
- ⬥ ¼ C olive oil or melted lard
- ⬥ 1 tsp salt
- ⬥ Zest of one lemon, about 1 tsp

INSTRUCTIONS AND HOW KIDS CAN HELP

1. Cut or tear kale off of thick stems, into 2-inch squares (approximately bite size).
2. Toss with olive oil or lard, salt, and lemon zest.
3. Lay out cut kale onto baking sheet in a single non-overlapping layer.
4. Roast at 400 degrees for 15 minutes until crispy, stirring every 5 minutes.

Preheat oven to
170 degrees

Special Tools:
Mandolin (optional),
Dehydrator (optional
but recommended).

Notes:

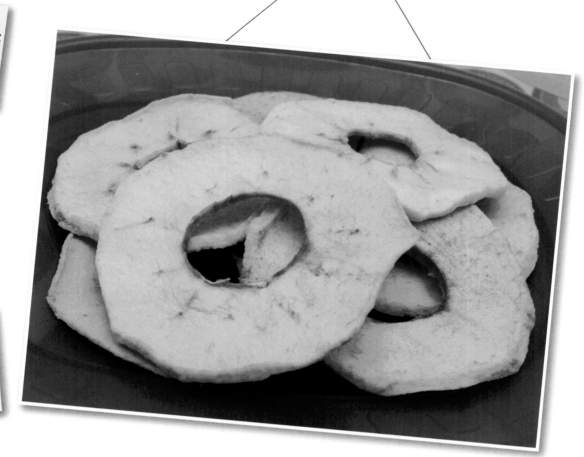

164

Eat Like a Dinosaur

APPLE RINGS

Makes about 50 rings

You know what's more delicious than an apple? Apples that don't have a core or ever get bruised. We make these apple rings so we can snack on apples without getting sticky all the time. Put them in your lunch or keep some in the car for the next time you get really hungry but aren't close to home. We bet you can't eat just one!

INGREDIENTS

- ◊ 4 large apples (a mild flavor like Fuji, York, or Gala works best)

INSTRUCTIONS AND HOW KIDS CAN HELP

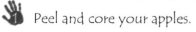 Peel and core your apples.

2. Carefully slice apples into rings 1/8 inch to 1/4 inch thick with either a knife or mandolin. The thinner the more crispy the apple ring—your preference, but we like ours about 1/4 inch thick so they have a little chew to them.

3. Dry in dehydrator on medium heat for 6 to 12 hours (apples should be dry yet flexible) or bake in oven in single layers on baking sheets at 170 degrees for 12-24 hours, checking for firmness.

Preheat oven to 170 degrees

Special Tools:
Dehydrator
(optional but
recommended)

Notes:

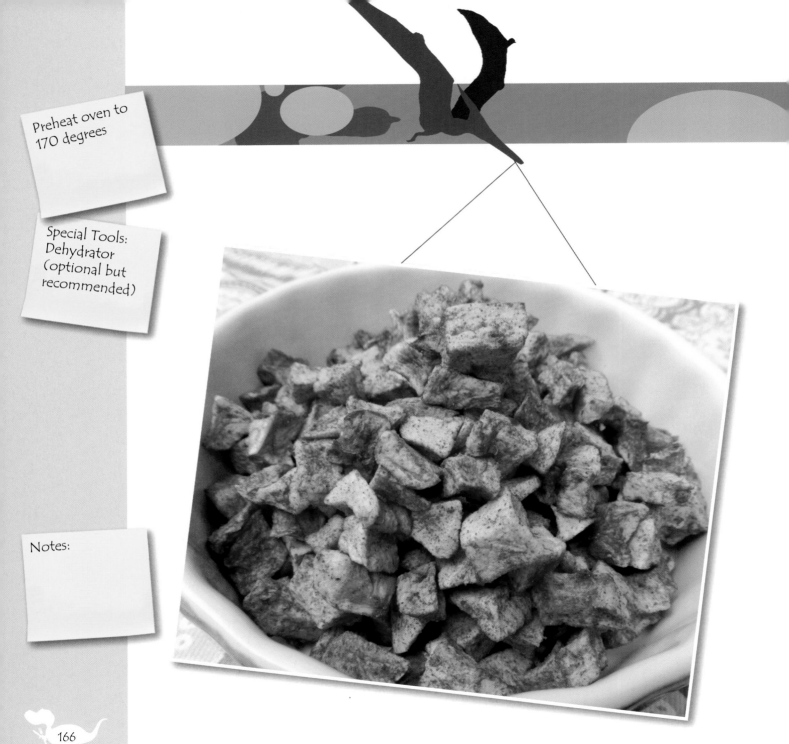

Eat Like a Dinosaur

CINNAMON APPLE TIDBITS

Makes a quart of apple tidbits

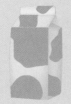

This recipe is just like our Apple Rings (p. 165), only it adds cinnamon and makes the apple pieces into little tidbits, perfect for munching on and adding to trail mixes. With the addition of cinnamon, these are deliciously tasty.

We like this recipe even more than the apple rings, simply because we can make more apples in less time with our dehydrator. If you're using an oven, make sure that the apples don't overlap or they won't be able to properly dry out.

INGREDIENTS

- ◇ 5 large apples (a mild flavor like Fuji, York, or Gala)
- ◇ 1 Tbsp cinnamon

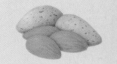

INSTRUCTIONS AND HOW KIDS CAN HELP

1. Peel and core your apples.

2. Dice apples into ¼-inch pieces (lay out the pieces on the tray or baking sheet as you go so that you know how many apples to dice; each of our trays fit about 4 large apples).

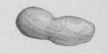

3. Toss the apples with cinnamon until coated.

4. Dry in dehydrator on medium heat for up to 4 hours until apple bits are dry on the outside yet still spongy and flexible on the inside.

5. Alternatively, bake in oven on a baking sheet at 170 degrees for 6–8 hours, checking for firmness.

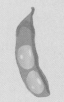

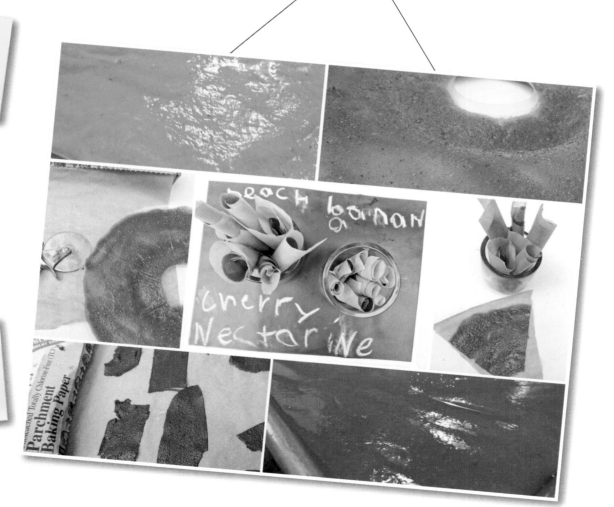

Eat Like a Dinosaur

ROLLED FRUIT LEATHERS

Makes 12 servings

CHERRY NECTARINE

- ◇ 4 ripe nectarines
- ◇ 2 C cherries, pitted
- ◇ ¾ C water
- ◇ 1 Tbsp almond extract

You probably love fruit snacks. I know we did. Fruit snacks were one of the things we were very sad to find out wasn't really a food a dinosaur would eat, since the store brands have lots of sugar and chemicals in them. What we learned is that you can make them at home in a much healthier way!

This roll up flavor is tangy like a cherry, and a fun and natural bright red. This is definitely a snack you might catch your parents eating when you're not looking! And since you can store these almost anywhere, it's a great snack to keep in the car, sports bag, or snack box for school.

PEACH BANANA

- ◇ 4 peaches, very ripe
- ◇ 2 ripe bananas
- ◇ ¾ C water
- ◇ 1 Tbsp vanilla

This roll up flavor is made with bananas and peaches and is very sweet and flavorful. Out of all the kinds we've made, this is Cole's absolute favorite.

Ask your farmer for a discount on a big box of fruit; bruised and over ripe fruit are perfect for this recipe.

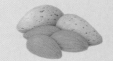

INSTRUCTIONS AND HOW KIDS CAN HELP

1. Blanch stone fruit in pot of boiling water for 2–3 minutes.
2. Immediately place fruit in an ice water bath.
3. Peel skin off, cut in half, and remove pits.
4. Place peeled halves with other fruit and water in medium sauce pan and bring to boil over medium heat.
5. Reduce heat to low and simmer for 30 minutes, using a potato masher every 5–10 minutes to break up and soften the fruit.
6. When finished cooking, add flavor extract and blend until smooth.
7. Pour onto baking sheet lined with a silicone mat or plastic wrap (we recommend the plastic sheet of your dehydrator if you have one).
8. Use a spatula to add thickness to the edges—the edges will dry too fast if they are not slightly thicker than the center (slightly thicken about 30% of the width at the edges).
9. Bake at 170 degrees for 10–12 hours (watch your pan as you near the finish, your edges may finish cooking first) or dehydrate for 8 hours.
10. Use a pizza cutter to segment the fruit leather into the size of your choosing.
11. Lay out on parchment or wax paper, roll up, and store in an airtight container.

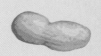

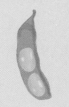

Notes:

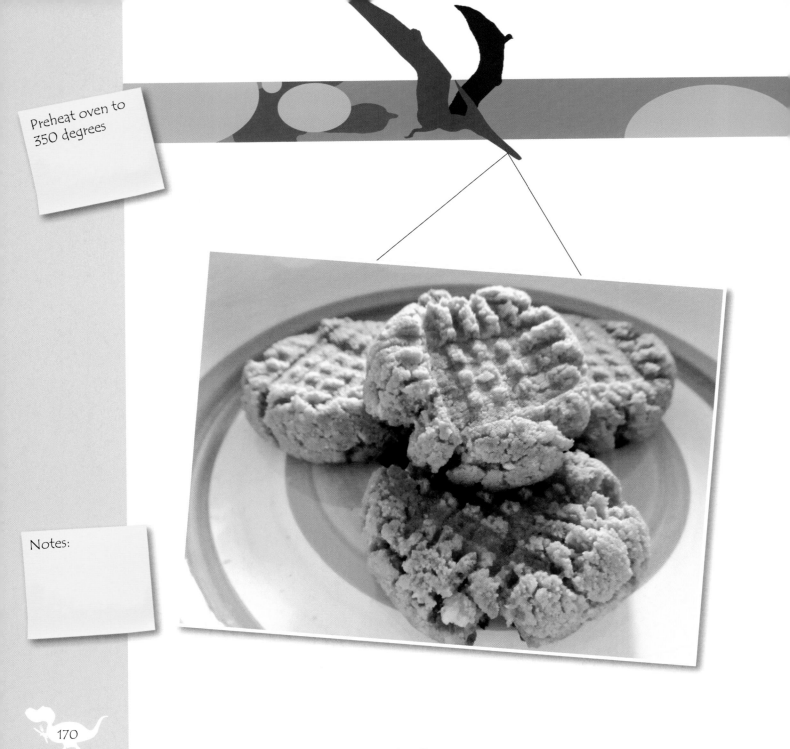

170

Eat Like a Dinosaur

ANYTIME COOKIES

Makes 24 cookies

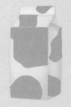

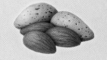
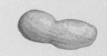

A certain blue-furred monster has been known to say that cookies are a "sometimes" food. Normally that's absolutely true, except in our house we make cookies entirely out of healthy foods and eat them anytime! They remind us of a flavorful shortbread (or peanut butter) cookie. They're so good you'll want them for your snack.

We like to add blueberries, chopped nuts, dates, raisins, and all kinds of other ingredients. Make them plain or add your favorite flavorings, and pack one in your next lunchbox !

INGREDIENTS

- 1 banana, peeled
- 1 apple, cored and peeled
- ½ C almond butter (crunchy preferred)
- 3 Tbsp palm shortening or butter
- 1 Tbsp vanilla
- 1½ C almond flour
- 1 tsp baking soda
- ½ tsp salt
- ½ C of your favorite ingredient (Optional)

INSTRUCTIONS AND HOW KIDS CAN HELP

1. Purée banana and apple together in a food processor.
2. Add purée, almond butter, shortening, and vanilla to bowl and beat until combined.
3. In separate bowl, mix together flour, baking soda, and salt.
4. Add dry ingredients to wet and mix until dough forms.
5. Form into tablespoon-sized balls and place on greased or lined cookie sheet (press with a fork in opposite directions for a pretty design).
6. Bake at 350 degrees for 8 to 12 minutes.
7. Store in an airtight container at room temperature for up to a day or two, otherwise store refrigerated or in the freezer.

Notes:

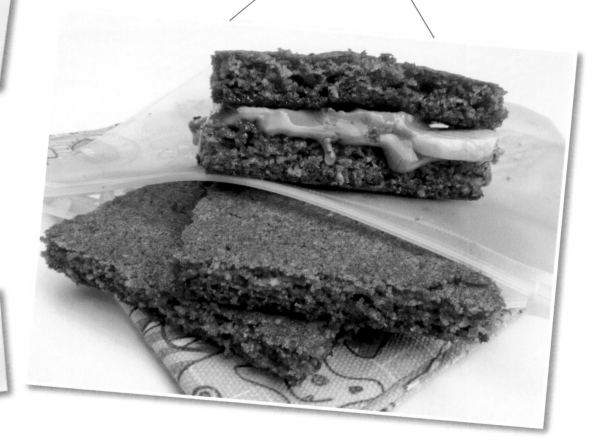

Eat Like a Dinosaur

GRAHAM COOKIES

Makes 24 cookies

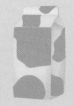

Since our boys sometimes missed sandwiches, we thought it'd be fun to make a "cookie" that was similar to a graham cracker AND bread! We love filling these with sunflower seed butter, honey, and banana slices for delicious sandwiches. We also love topping them with apple butter and placing them next to our eggs for breakfast.

We feel like we've even improved on your plain old box of crackers with these thick, bread-like cookies. You can use a cookie cutter with them to make fun shapes, and you can even make a graham pie crust by pulsing half your cooked cookies with three tablespoons of melted coconut oil!

INGREDIENTS

⋄ 1 C coconut flour	⋄ ½ C coconut oil, melted
⋄ ¾ C almond flour	⋄ ¼ C palm shortening or butter
⋄ ½ C tapioca flour	⋄ ¼ C unrefined granulated sugar
⋄ 2 tsp baking powder	⋄ 1 Tbsp vanilla extract
⋄ 2 tsp cinnamon	⋄ ¼ C honey
⋄ ½ tsp salt	⋄ 3 eggs

INSTRUCTIONS AND HOW KIDS CAN HELP

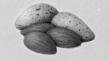 1. In a bowl, sift together the flours, baking powder, cinnamon, and salt.

2. Beat coconut oil, shortening, and sugar with an electric beater or stand mixer.

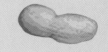 3. While mixing on low, add vanilla, honey, and eggs one at a time until just combined.

4. Slowly beat the dry ingredients into wet until dough forms; use a spatula to scrape edges and combine well.

 5. Spread dough onto a lined cookie sheet (silicone or parchment paper).

6. Bake for 10 minutes at 350 degrees, watching carefully so as not to burn.

 7. Cut with a pizza cutter or knife into the desired square size or use cookie cutters to make fun shapes.

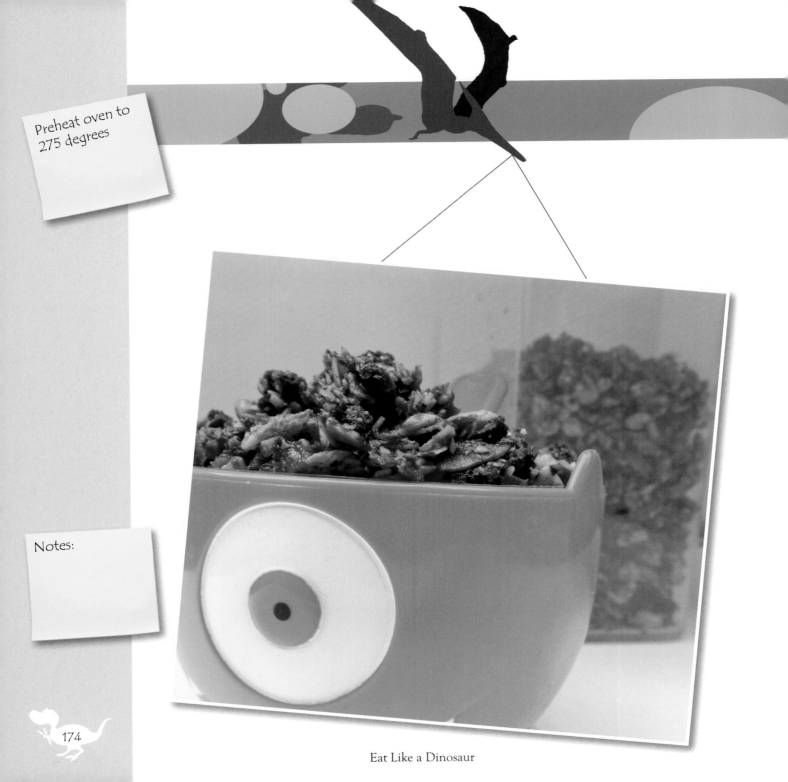

Preheat oven to 275 degrees

Notes:

Eat Like a Dinosaur

GRAIN-FREE GRANOLA
Makes 6 cups of granola

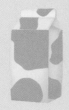

Having changed what you eat, you probably miss cereal from time to time. We're not going to lie: we miss cereal, too. Granola has always been a favorite, but with the traditional variety containing oats, we have to pass it up at the store. The good news is that this recipe tastes just like a granola cereal, and it's perfect with a bowl of coconut or other milk!

Give this recipe a shot; we think you'll love the nutty and crisp texture of this granola. Once you're good at making it, mix up the flavors and nuts with ingredients you love. Our boys have really love dried cranberries, but raisins or any variety of dried fruit would work well. Maybe you'd prefer pecans instead of walnuts. Anyway you'd like it, we think you'll love eating granola again!

INGREDIENTS

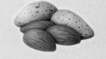

- 1½ C sliced almonds
- 1½ C coconut flakes, chopped
- 1 C walnuts, chopped finely or puréed into a meal
- 1 C macadamia nuts, chopped finely or puréed into a meal
- 1 C dried cranberries
- ½ C fresh medjool dates, chopped to same size as cranberries
- ½ C coconut oil, melted (extra for greasing pan)
- ⅓ C honey
- 2 tsp cinnamon

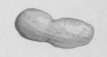

INSTRUCTIONS AND HOW KIDS CAN HELP

1. Combine almonds, coconut flakes, nuts, and fruit in a bowl.
2. Whisk together oil, honey, and cinnamon.
3. Pour oil-honey mixture over nuts and fruit, then mix.
4. Spread onto a WELL-greased baking sheet.
5. Bake for one hour at 275 degrees, stirring every 15 minutes to prevent burning.
6. Store in airtight container at room temperature for up to several months.

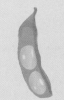

Preheat oven to
250 degrees

Notes:

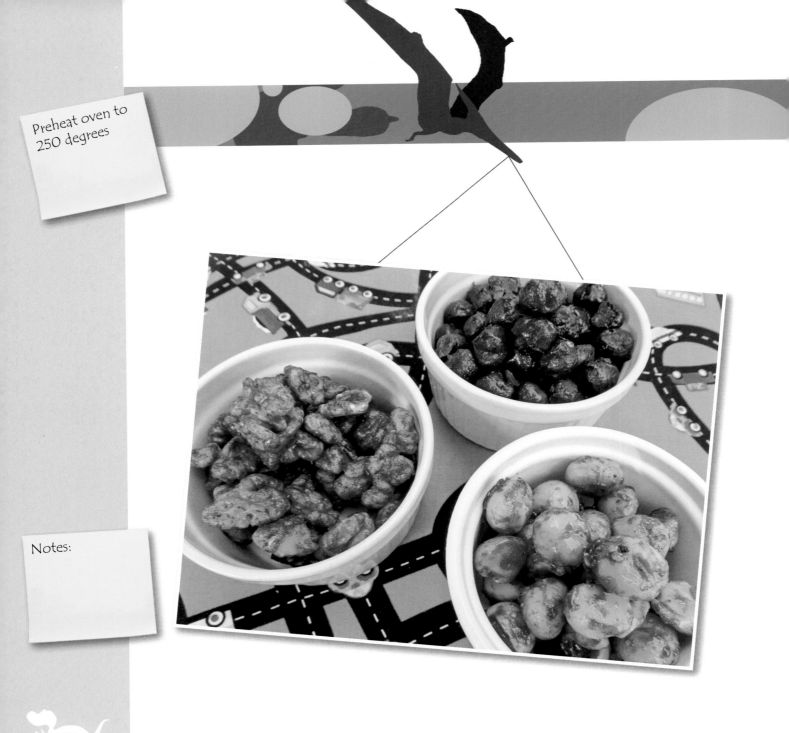

Eat Like a Dinosaur

CANDIED NUTS

Makes 2 cups each

CHOCOLATE-COVERED HAZELNUTS

- ◊ 2 C raw hazelnuts
- ◊ ¼ C Caramel Sauce (p. 243), room temperature
- ◊ 1 Tbsp cocoa powder
- ◊ ⅛ tsp salt
- ◊ Coconut oil to grease baking sheet

We love Nutella! It's a spread made with chocolate and hazelnuts. Baking cocoa hazelnuts this way has the same flavor we loved but with much less sugar. Plus, the crunch of the real hazelnuts is perfect for snacking!

If you're REALLY missing a chocolate hazelnut spread, simply grind the chocolate hazelnuts up into a paste with unsweetened almond milk—yum!

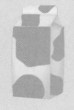

SWEET SPICED WALNUTS

- ◊ 2 C raw walnuts
- ◊ ¼ C Caramel Sauce (p. 243), room temperature
- ◊ ½ tsp cinnamon
- ◊ ¼ tsp salt
- ◊ ⅛ tsp nutmeg
- ◊ Coconut oil to grease baking sheet

Walnuts are one of our favorite nuts because they look like little brains! What's great is that this nut has Omega-3s, a healthy fat for your brain! We bake our walnuts with this sweet spice mix for a neat snack that has a little extra flavor. It goes great in a trail mix or simply snack on it whenever you'd like!

CARAMELIZED MACADAMIA NUTS

- ◊ 2 C raw macadamia nuts
- ◊ ¼ C Caramel Sauce (p. 243), room temperature
- ◊ ¼ tsp cinnamon
- ◊ ¼ tsp ground cumin
- ◊ ⅛ tsp ground cloves
- ◊ ⅛ tsp salt
- ◊ Coconut oil to grease baking sheet

Macadamia nuts are little round nuts from Hawaii that we feel are probably the healthiest and tastiest nut you can find! We use some surprising spices on them in this recipe. We love the unique flavor and think they're guaranteed tasty!

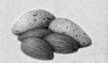
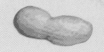

INSTRUCTIONS AND HOW KIDS CAN HELP

1. Grease baking sheet well.
2. Combine nuts, caramel, and spices on oiled baking sheet.
3. Toss and mix until well coated.
4. Roast in 250-degree oven for 45 minutes.
5. Store at room temperature for up to several weeks.

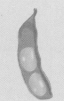

177

Snacks

Notes:

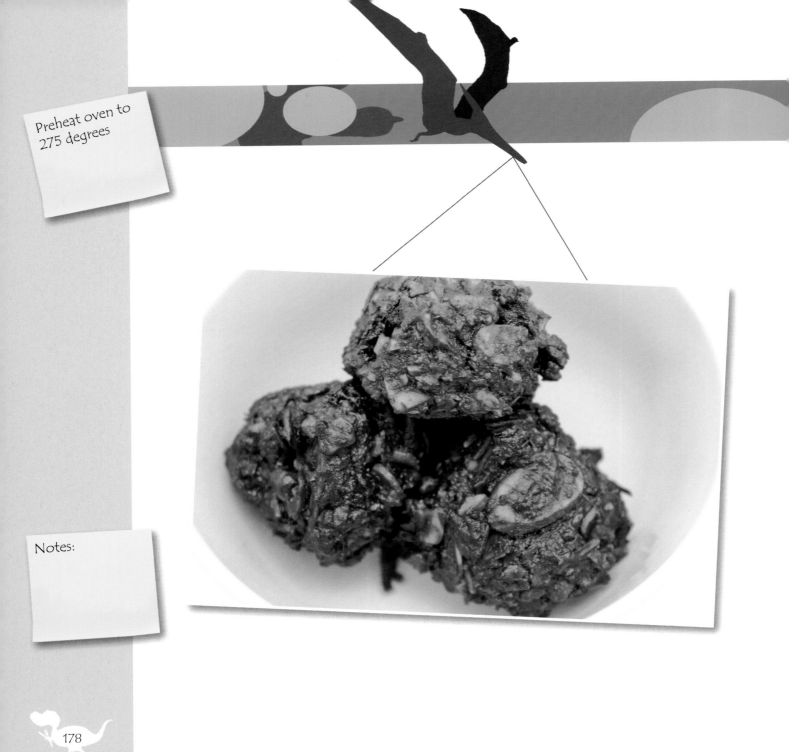

Eat Like a Dinosaur

CHERRY CHOCOLATE BALLS

Makes about 24 balls

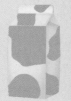

One of our favorite activities is picking fruit from our local "u-pick" farm. When cherries are ripe, we always pick lots and lots of them because it's fun to climb trees and it's nice and shady picking. We pit them, freeze them, and use them all year long in smoothies and recipes.

These snacks use the cherries we pick and freeze, but you can get yours at the store if you don't have any from a farm. Cherry Chocolate Balls are a super-yummy cross between a granola bar and cake balls.

INGREDIENTS

- ⋄ ⅔ C fresh or dried dates, rehydrated
- ⋄ ⅓ C cocoa powder
- ⋄ ¼ C honey
- ⋄ ½ C macadamia nuts
- ⋄ ⅓ C pecans
- ⋄ 1 C sliced almonds
- ⋄ 1 C pitted cherries, thawed from frozen and chopped

INSTRUCTIONS AND HOW KIDS CAN HELP

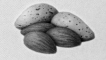

1. To rehydrate dried dates, cover with boiling water for 15 minutes, then strain.
2. Add dates, cocoa powder, and honey to food processor and purée; set aside.
3. In a clean food processor, pulse macadamia and pecan nuts into a fine grainy texture, pour mixture into bowl with set-aside wet ingredients.
4. Fold sliced almonds and chopped cherries into batter, mixing thoroughly.
5. Roll out 1½ inch balls and place on greased (or lined) baking sheet.
6. Bake at 275 degrees for 30 minutes.
7. Flip each ball and return to oven for 20–30 minutes until balls are firm.

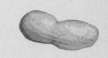

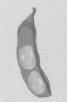

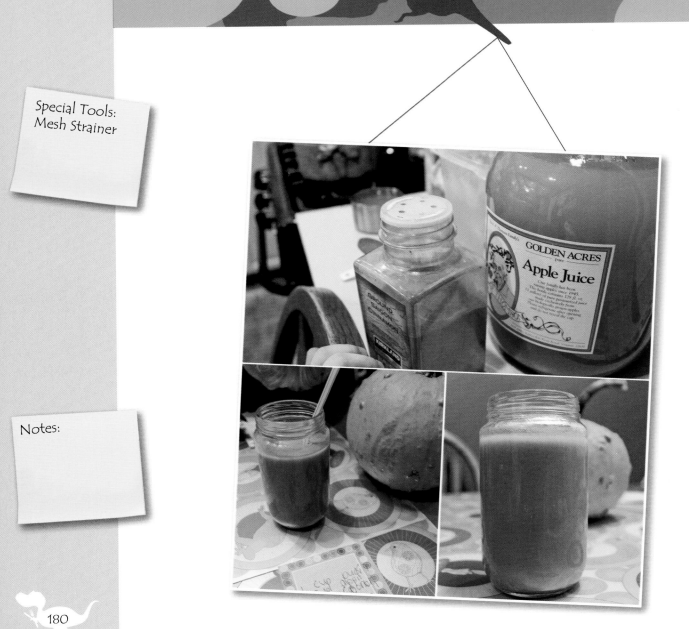

Eat Like a Dinosaur

Pumpkin Cider "Latte"

Serves 4

One cool fall morning we woke up and decided we needed a warm drink to get us through the day. Cole came up with the idea to make his very own version of a winter drink using some pumpkin and apple juice. The boys loved pretending they were drinking coffee, so we named it after a popular coffee drink that grown-ups have.

Ingredients

- ◊ 1 C pumpkin purée
- ◊ 1 C pure apple juice or cider
- ◊ 1 C boxed or light canned coconut milk
- ◊ 1 tsp ground cinnamon or 1 cinnamon stick
- ◊ ¼ tsp ground nutmeg

Instructions and How Kids Can Help

1. In a medium saucepan, whisk together the pumpkin, juice, and milk over medium heat.

2. If using cinnamon stick, add to pot.

3. Simmer until it just begins to boil while constantly stirring, about 10 minutes.

4. Whisk in powered spices until combined and remove from heat.

5. Strain and server warm; store for up to several weeks.

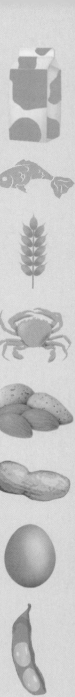

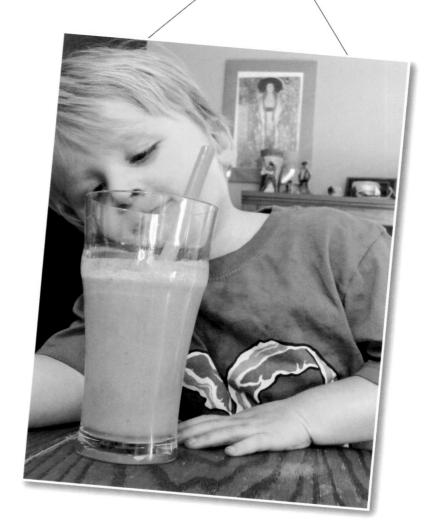

Eat Like a Dinosaur

Elvis's Nut Butter and Nana Smoothie

Makes 16 oz of smoothie

When we make this smoothie, one of us will do the full lip curl and explain to the kids that we're making an "almond butter and 'nana smoothie." Grown-ups think this is funny because there used to be a famous singer that said things like that, and nut butter with banana was one of his favorite foods. This smoothie is one of our favorites too, and it's so easy to make!

INGREDIENTS

- ◇ 1½ C unsweetened vanilla almond or hemp milk
- ◇ 1 ripe banana, peeled and frozen
- ◇ 3 Tbsp almond butter
- ◇ 1 Tbsp honey (optional, not needed if banana is super ripe)

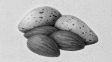

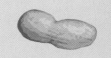

 ## INSTRUCTIONS AND HOW KIDS CAN HELP

1 Combine all ingredients in a blender and blend until smooth.

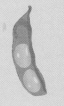

Notes:

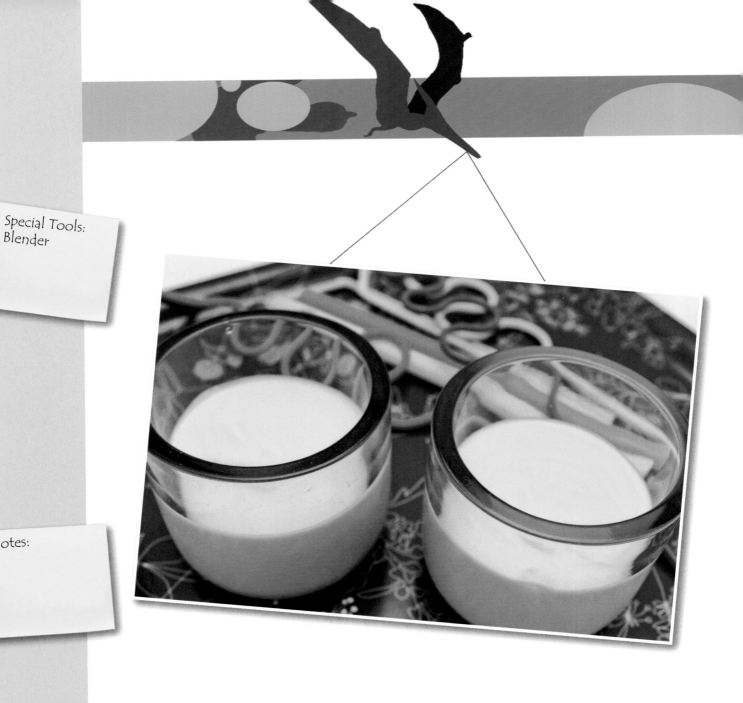

Eat Like a Dinosaur

HAWAIIAN VACATION SMOOTHIE

Makes 16 oz smoothie

Sometimes, especially in the cold of winter, it's fun to use your imagination and pretend you're on vacation. Use tropical fruits like mango and pineapple to make a "vacation smoothie" like this one. Then put on your bathing suit and sunglasses and pretend you're on a tropical island beach, sipping this treat through a straw. It's delicious, and the healthy fats in the coconut milk and macadamia nuts will keep you nourished for quite a while!

If you use fresh fruit instead of frozen, then replace half the water with ice to make this a nice, cool smoothie.

INGREDIENTS

- ◇ ¼ C raw macadamia nuts
- ◇ 1 C coconut milk
- ◇ ½ C ice or water
- ◇ ½ C fresh or frozen mangos
- ◇ ½ C fresh or frozen pineapples

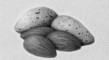

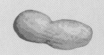

INSTRUCTIONS AND HOW KIDS CAN HELP

 In blender, pulse nuts until they are the consistency of sand.

Add remaining ingredients and purée until smooth.

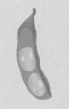

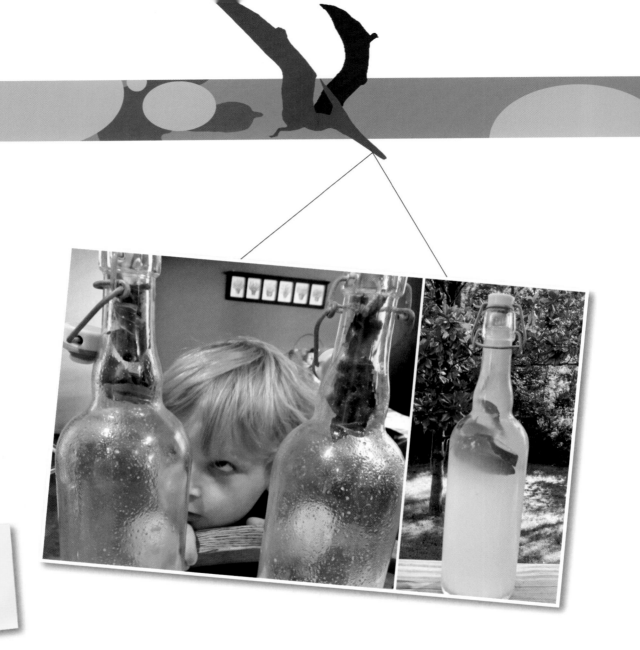

Eat Like a Dinosaur

PINEAPPLE, MINT, AND CLEMENTINE WATER

Makes one gallon

We love pineapple, so we're always looking for something to do with the leftover juice when we use canned pineapple in our recipes. We found that mixing it with water, fresh mint, and clementine creates a fresh, fruity, and fun drink that's perfectly refreshing when you're looking for something a bit more special than regular water. If you don't have a clementine at home, you can also use lemon, lime, or orange!

INGREDIENTS

- ◇ 1 C pineapple juice (remaining liquid of 16 oz can)
- ◇ 24–40 fresh mint leaves, washed
- ◇ 1 clementine
- ◇ 56 oz water (approximate)

INSTRUCTIONS AND HOW KIDS CAN HELP

1. Add the pineapple juice and mint to a clean pitcher.
2. Zest and juice the clementine; add to pitcher.
3. Fill the rest of the pitcher with water.
4. Let little hands stir, muddle, or shake.
5. Serve cold.

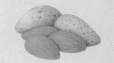
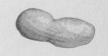

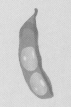

What we like to do in our house is call dessert a "special treat." It's not something we have every day, and when we do, we eat a small amount and really enjoy how delicious it tastes. Your brain might sometimes tell you that you should have more, but that's because your tricky little taste buds are telling your brain it tastes good. If you're still hungry, choose something from one of the other sections of this book.

The thing about sweets is that they're treats. No matter what kind of ingredients you use, something sweet will have sugar in it, and even natural sugars can make your body behave a little funny. The recipes in this section are healthier than other desserts because we use natural and unrefined sweeteners, like dates, honey, and maple syrup. Of course, they're grain and dairy-free too.

It's funny to imagine a dinosaur wearing a birthday party hat and eating cake, isn't it? We don't think dinosaurs could even bake a muffin, let alone a whole cake! So, use the big human brain you have to help you save and choose your special treats for special occasions!

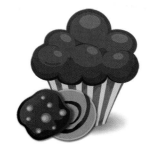

CHAPTER 7
SPECIAL TREATS

Preheat oven to
350 degrees

Special Tools:
Electric mixer or
stand mixer

Notes:

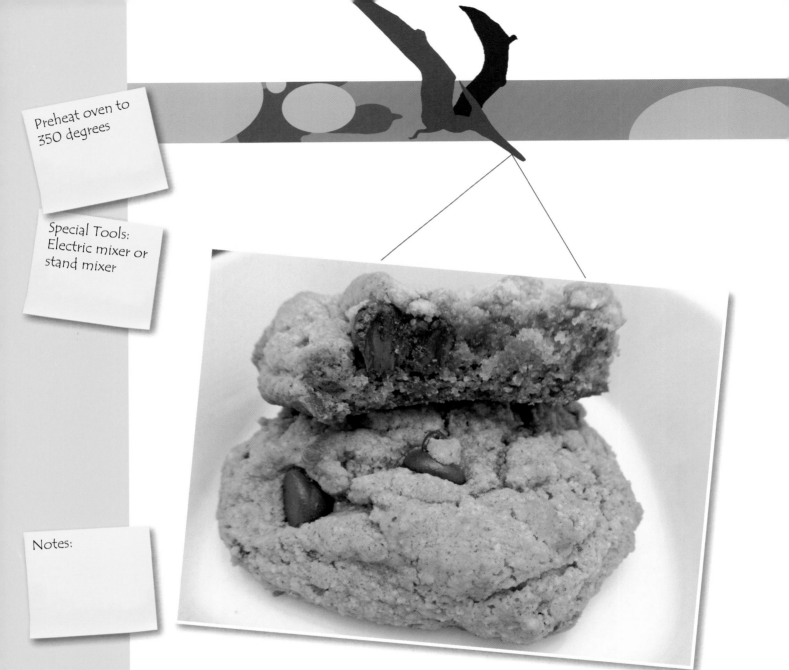

Eat Like a Dinosaur

CHOCOLATE CHIP COOKIES

Makes 24 cookies

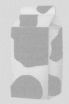

These chocolate chip cookies are amazingly delicious. As a matter of fact, we think they're even better than any chocolate chip cookie we had before we ate like dinosaurs. We like to dip ours in (unsweetened) chocolate almond milk, but they're also great on their own. We're always finding the boys with chocolate mustaches when we have a batch in the house.

INGREDIENTS

- ½ C palm shortening or butter
- ½ C dates, chopped finely
- ¼ C honey
- 2 eggs
- 2 Tbsp vanilla extract
- 2 C almond flour
- 1 tsp baking soda
- ½ tsp salt
- ½ C chocolate chips

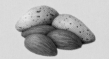

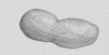

INSTRUCTIONS AND HOW KIDS CAN HELP

1. Cream together shortening, dates, and honey using electric or stand mixer.
2. Scrape the side of the mixing bowl, then add eggs and vanilla and beat to combine.
3. In a separate bowl, combine flour, baking soda, and salt.
4. Add dry mixture to wet and beat until just combined.
5. Fold in chocolate chips.
6. Spoon a heaping tablespoon for each cookie onto greased or lined baking sheet.
7. Bake for 8–10 minutes at 350 degrees.
8. Store chilled for a week or more.

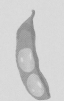

Special Treats

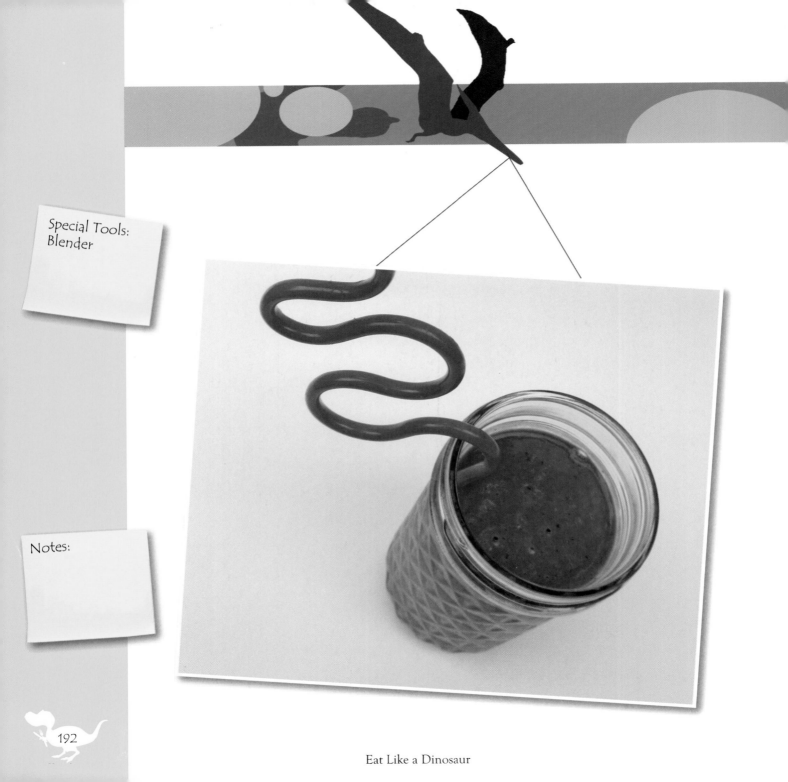

Special Tools:
Blender

Notes:

192

Chocolate Milkshake

Serves 2-4

We love avocados in our family and try to put them in EVERYTHING. What better way to add smooth, rich flavor to a drink than adding a whole avocado to it? This smoothie is so creamy and thick, we've started calling it a milkshake!

INGREDIENTS

- 2 dates, fresh or rehydrated
- 1 (14 oz) can full-fat coconut milk (chilled)
- 1 C ice
- 1 avocado, skin and pit removed
- 1 ripe banana, frozen
- ¼ C cocoa powder

INSTRUCTIONS AND HOW KIDS CAN HELP

1. To rehydrate dates, cover with boiling water for 15 minutes.
2. Combine all ingredients in blender and purée until smooth.
3. Results in a particularly thick, rich, and delicious treat!

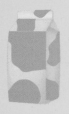

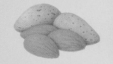
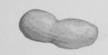

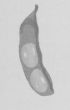

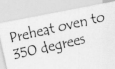

Preheat oven to 350 degrees

Special Tools:
Electric mixer or stand mixer

Notes:

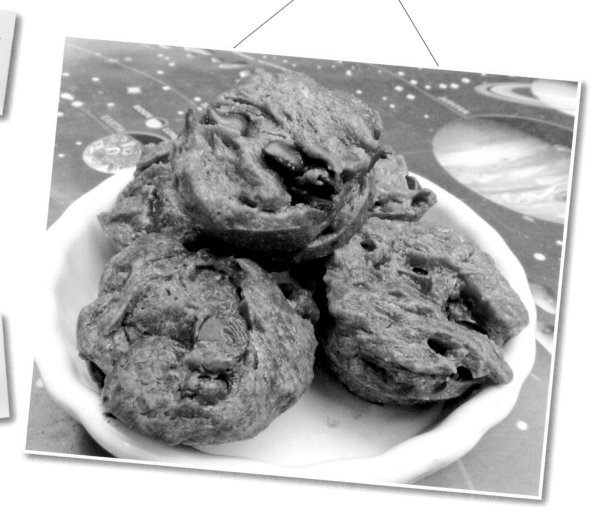

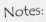

194

Eat Like a Dinosaur

MINI NUT BUTTER CUPS

Makes 24 mini cups or 9 muffin size

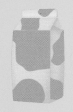
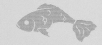

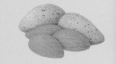
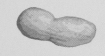

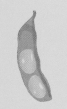

These mini muffins taste like a peanut butter candy walked into a muffin, only they're much healthier. If you've never tried sunflower seed butter before, you're in for a treat! It's the seeds of a sunflower ground up like peanut butter.

INGREDIENTS

- ⋄ 2 eggs
- ⋄ 1 overripe, mashed banana
- ⋄ 1 C sunflower seed butter (we recommend SunButter or Trader Joe's brand)
- ⋄ ½ tsp sea salt
- ⋄ ½ C mini chocolate chips
- ⋄ ⅓ C chopped pecans (Optional)

INSTRUCTIONS AND HOW KIDS CAN HELP

1. Beat eggs and banana together.
2. Once combined, beat in sunflower seed butter and salt.
3. Fold in chocolate chips and pecans.
4. Bake at 350 degrees for 8–10 minutes for mini muffins or 13–15 minutes for regular size. (Bubbling oil on the edges from sunflower seed butter may make them appear not done; take them out and let them cool once the middle is not spongy.)
5. Store chilled for a week or more.

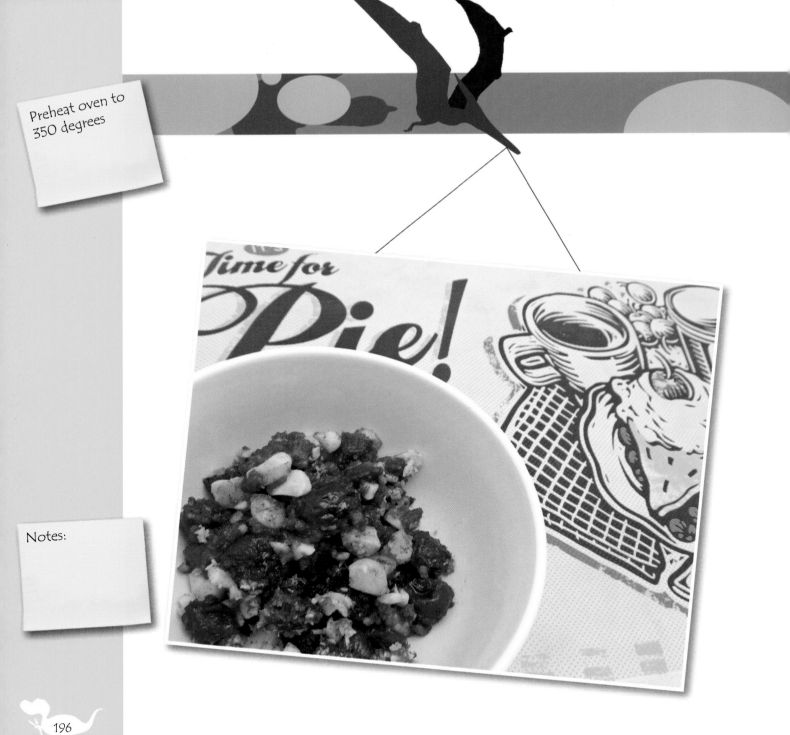

Preheat oven to 350 degrees

Notes:

196

Eat Like a Dinosaur

CHERRY MACADAMIA CRUMBLE

Serves 10

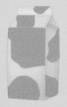

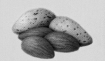
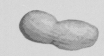

We love cherry picking! After climbing the trees and picking these little cute gems, making this delicious dessert is the perfect way to end the day. It's even better with our Honey Nut Ice Cream (p. 237) on top!

We use a cherry pitter (we got ours at the dollar store) to remove the seeds of the cherries when we get home from the farm. Then we freeze them for summer-fresh cherries all year long!

INGREDIENTS

- 5 C frozen tart cherries
- ¾ C dates, diced finely and separated
- ½ C maple syrup
- ¼ C palm shortening or butter
- 2 Tbsp honey
- 2 eggs
- 1 Tbsp vanilla extract
- 1 C coconut flour
- 1 C raw macadamia nuts, chopped
- 1 Tbsp and 1 tsp cinnamon, separated
- 1 tsp baking soda
- ½ tsp salt
- ½ C coconut oil
- ½ tsp nutmeg

INSTRUCTIONS AND HOW KIDS CAN HELP

1. Combine cherries, ½ cup dates, and maple syrup in mixing bowl—be sure to break up any date or cherry clumps.
2. Spread cherry mixture into greased 9-by-13-inch baking dish.
3. Beat palm shortening, ¼ cup dates, and honey together.
4. Add eggs and whip until thoroughly combined.
5. In separate bowl, whisk together flour, macadamia nuts, 1 tablespoon of cinnamon, baking soda, and salt.
6. Slowly add mixed dry ingredients into wet until a crumbly mixture forms.
7. Sprinkle crumble over cherry mixture in the baking dish.
8. Mix coconut oil with remaining teaspoon of cinnamon and nutmeg; drizzle over top of crumble.
9. Bake at 350 degrees for 45–60 minutes (fresh cherries may take longer than 45 minutes).

Special Treats

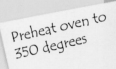

Preheat oven to 350 degrees

Special Tools: Food processor or blender

Notes:

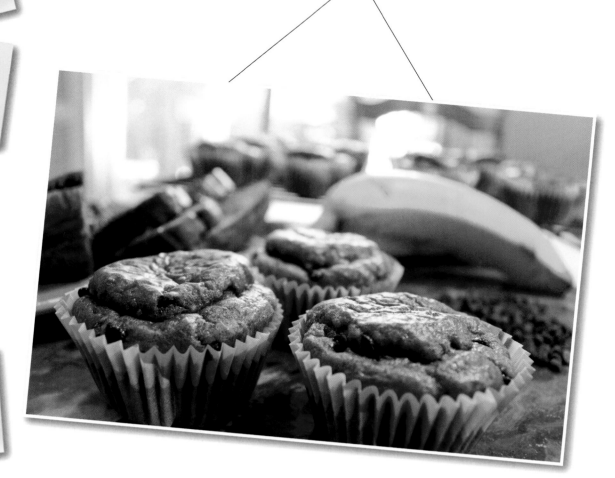

198

BANANA CHOCOLATE CHIP BREAD

Makes 1 loaf or 15 muffins

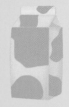

Not often, but sometimes, your bananas get overripe before you eat them. Don't let them go to waste because of a few freckles or bruises! You can freeze them for use in our Hawaiian Vacation Smoothie (p. 185) or you can make this wonderful warm and moist banana bread. We promise it's so good you might even let your next bananas get overripe on purpose so you can make it again!

INGREDIENTS

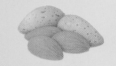
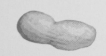

◊ 1 C almond butter (or MaraNatha brand sunflower butter)	◊ 1 tsp cinnamon
◊ 4 eggs	◊ ½ tsp baking soda
◊ 1 overripe banana, chunked	◊ ¼ tsp salt
	◊ ⅓ C mini chocolate chips

INSTRUCTIONS AND HOW KIDS CAN HELP

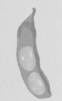

1. In food processor or blender, purée all ingredients except chocolate chips together until smooth, scraping the side of the bowl to incorporate all of the nut butter into the batter (some small banana pieces may remain).
2. Fold chocolate chips into batter gently with a spoon or spatula.
3. Pour into greased (we use Spectrum coconut oil spray) loaf or scoop ¼ cup batter into each cup of muffin pan.
4. Bake at 350 degrees for 30 minutes for a small loaf pan or 15-18 minutes for muffins.
5. Store chilled for a week or more.

199

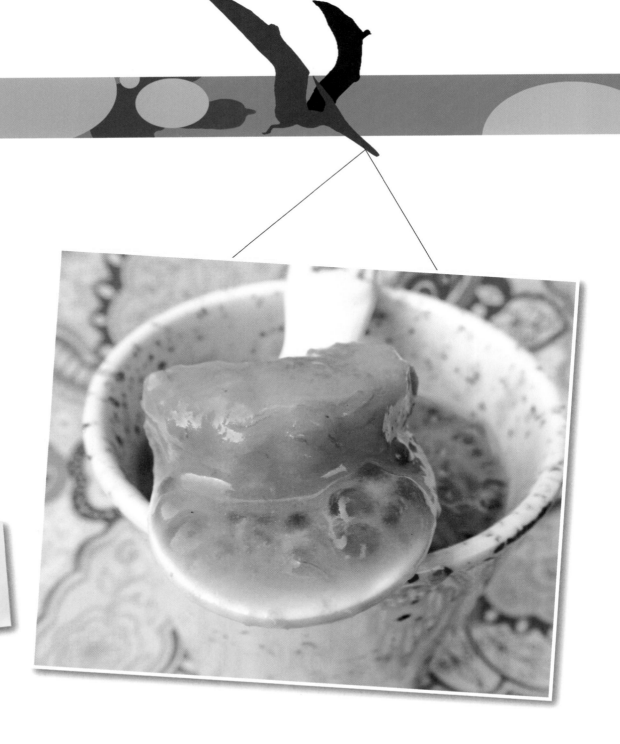

Notes:

Eat Like a Dinosaur

BANANA BUBBLE PUDDING

Provides 10–12 servings

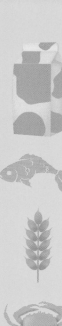

Tapioca pearls look like hundreds of tiny bubbles when you cook them, but really they're just tiny balls of starch made from the cassava root. We add them to pudding and, voila, bubble pudding!

Tapioca pearls can be found affordably and easily at any Asian food market if you are unable to find them at your local grocery store. A little bit goes a long way, so if you're like us and can never eat enough bananas, try this pudding!

INGREDIENTS

- ⅓ C tapioca pearls (not instant tapioca)
- 6 bananas
- 1 (14 oz) can of full-fat coconut milk
- 1½ C water
- ⅓ C unrefined granulated sugar
- ¼ tsp salt

INSTRUCTIONS AND HOW KIDS CAN HELP

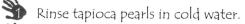

1. Rinse tapioca pearls in cold water.

2. Slice bananas into ½-inch half-rounds (or any bite-size shape the little hands choose).

3. Combine coconut milk, water, sugar, and salt in pot over medium heat.

4. Stir continuously for 2–3 minutes over medium heat, until sugar is dissolved.

5. Add rinsed tapioca pearls and bananas to milk mixture.

6. Check and stir occasionally while mixture cooks over medium heat (10–20 minutes).

7. Have little eyes watch to let you know once tapioca is translucent, and then remove from heat and let cool.

8. Serve hot or cold. Store in an airtight container in the refrigerator for up to two weeks.

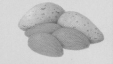
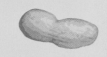

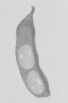

201

Special Tools:
Electric mixer or
stand mixer

Notes:

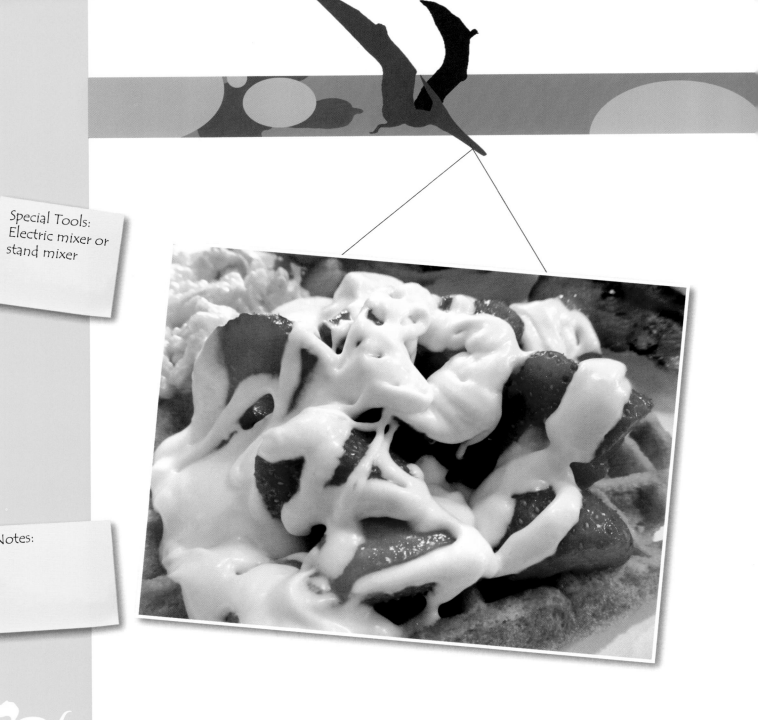

WHIPPED COCONUT CREAM

Makes 1 cup of whipped coconut cream

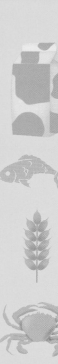

We love to put berries and coconut cream on our Sunday morning Frozen Waffles (p. 231), but they're also a delicious treat all by themselves. If you like to get the can of whipped cream from the fridge and spray it on your dessert, this is a great alternative with no dairy!

The coconut cream pairs well with all sorts of berries, but our favorites are strawberries and blueberries. It'd even be great on our Cherry Macadamia Crumble (p. 197)!

INGREDIENTS

- ◇ 1 (14 oz) can full-fat coconut milk, chilled in refrigerator overnight
- ◇ 2 Tbsp honey
- ◇ 1 pint of berries of your choice (optional)

INSTRUCTIONS AND HOW KIDS CAN HELP

1. Open can and scoop the thick white hardened cream into mixer (about 4 oz).
2. Beat on a medium to high setting for 2–3 minutes.
3. Add honey and beat for another 2–3 minutes, until cream thickens and becomes slightly stiff (it will not stand up like dairy whipped cream).
4. Serve immediately or store chilled for up to 2 weeks.

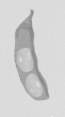

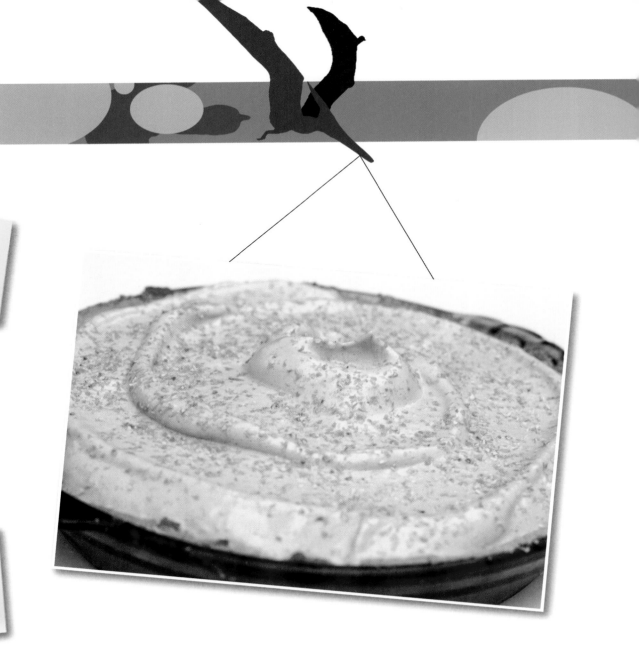

Special Tools:
Electric mixer or
stand mixer.
Strainer, colander
or cheesecloth.

Notes:

204

Coconut Cream Pie

Serves 8–10

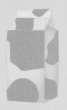

The first time we made coconut cream pie, we had a serious accident! We forgot to let the pie chill in the fridge, so when we tried to move it, it spilled everywhere! We made it again in hopes that it was tasty after all. Luckily, it's delicious and sets up nicely when you follow the directions!

The fun part of this recipe is in making the fluffy topping. As you whip the egg whites, the air begins to put bubbles in them and puffs them up.

Ingredients

◇ 2 C unsweetened vanilla almond milk	◇ 2 Tbsp coconut oil
◇ 1 C coconut milk	◇ 1 prebaked Pie Crust (p. 207)
◇ 1 Tbsp vanilla extract	◇ 4 egg whites, at room temperature
◇ 1½ C shredded unsweetened coconut	◇ ½ tsp cream of tartar
◇ ⅔ C unrefined granulated sugar	◇ ¼ C water
◇ 4 large egg yolks	◇ ½ C unrefined granulated sugar
◇ 6 Tbsp arrowroot powder	◇ ¼ C shredded unsweetened coconut, toasted
◇ ¼ tsp salt	

Instructions and How Kids Can Help

1. Combine almond milk, coconut milk, vanilla, and coconut in saucepan over medium heat until it just starts to bubble, about 5 minutes.
2. Remove from heat and cover for about 15 minutes.
3. In a separate bowl, whisk sugar, yolks, arrowroot, and salt together.
4. Strain milk mixture from coconut with strainer, colander, or cheesecloth.
5. Add strained milk slowly into yolk mixture while little hands whisk.
6. Return incorporated mixture to pot and bring to a boil over high heat.
7. Remove from heat and whisk in coconut oil until smooth.
8. Chill in refrigerator for ten minutes, then pour into prebaked pie crust.
9. Let set in the fridge for 2 hours.
10. When ready to serve, in a clean bowl, whip egg whites with tartar until soft peaks form.
11. In saucepan, whisk together water and sugar and bring to a boil over medium heat.
12. Continue boiling until thin syrup forms, about 6 minutes.
13. Start whipping eggs again while slowly dripping syrup into them until fully incorporated.
14. Spread on top of chilled pie, top with toasted coconut, and chill for up to 1 hour before eggs deflate.

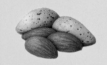
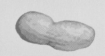

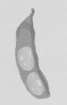

Special Treats

Notes:

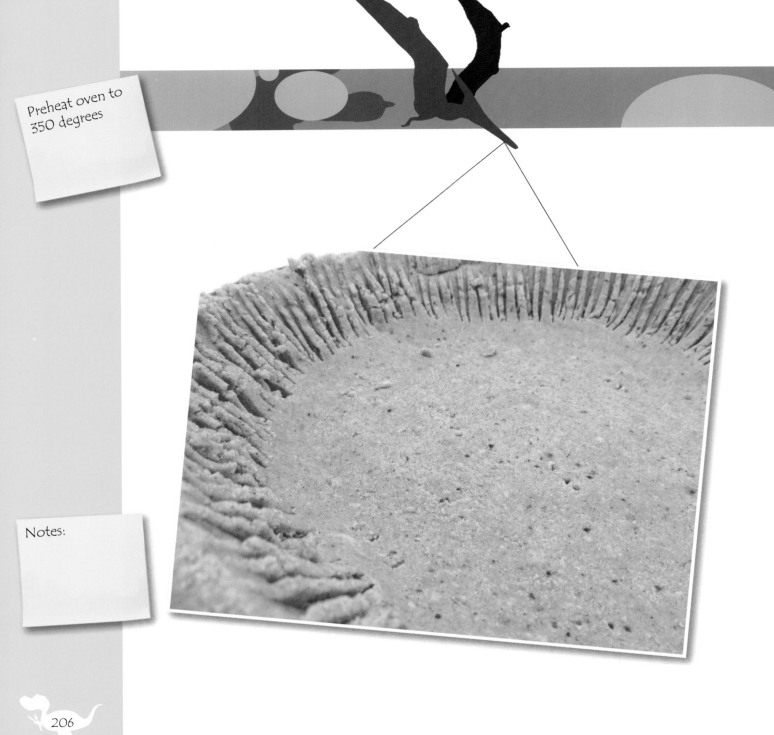

Eat Like a Dinosaur

PIE CRUST

Makes 1 pie crust

We've tried lots of different ways to make pie crusts and never found one to our liking. Some were too sweet, some were too flaky, some were even too difficult to make. One morning, Stacy woke up early and headed to the kitchen, determined to solve our pie crust dilemma. An hour later, she had invented a fantastic recipe! This is now our go-to crust.

INGREDIENTS

- 2 C almond flour
- ½ tsp baking soda
- ¼ tsp salt
- ½ C coconut oil, liquefied

INSTRUCTIONS AND HOW KIDS CAN HELP

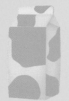

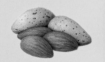
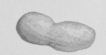

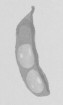

1. In a mixing bowl, sift together flour, soda, and salt.

2. Add oil and use fork to incorporate.

3. Press into pie pan gently, no higher than top of the pan—if you press too hard into the pan, the dough will not release easily once fully cooked; try to move the dough with the palm of your hand, rather than pushing down on the dough.

4. Pierce several times with a fork and "pretty" your edges.

5. Bake for 10–12 minutes at 350 degrees.

Notes:

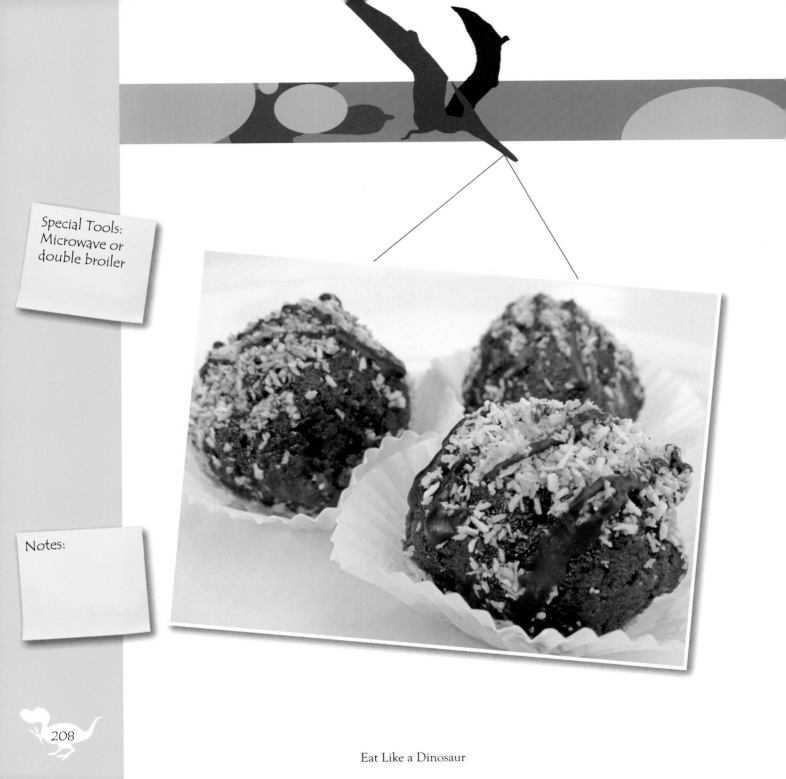

208

SAMOA CAKE BALLS

Makes 24 cake balls

We used to look forward to the Girl Scouts coming to our house so that we could purchase boxes of their Samoa cookies. This year when the young ladies came a-knockin', we (somewhat sadly) politely declined. The boys got to asking why they didn't have gluten-free options, and my only recourse was to figure out a way to bring the same flavors into our own kitchen.

Never fear, Samoa cake balls are here! These delicious bite-size treats are worth their effort and a huge hit with guests, too. They freeze really well and are a perfect make-ahead treat to save for when you have a party to attend and you'd like to bring your own treat to share.

INGREDIENTS

- ½ batch of our Red Brownie Cupcakes (p. 225)
- 1 batch Caramel Icing (p. 219)
- ½ C Caramel Sauce (p. 243)
- 1 C unsweetened shredded coconut, toasted and finely chopped
- 2 oz dark chocolate
- 1 Tbsp palm shortening or butter

INSTRUCTIONS AND HOW KIDS CAN HELP

1. Crumble cooled cake into bowl, spoon icing over top of cake bits and mix by hand to incorporate.

2. Form into balls of cake and gently place on parchment or wax paper to set in refrigerator or freezer for at least 30 minutes to firm.

3. Warm Caramel Sauce to bring to a liquid state and dip half of the cake ball into caramel sauce.

4. Immediately dip sticky caramel–side of cake ball into toasted coconut; set aside to repeat batch.

5. Melt chocolate with shortening in double boiler (make your own with a 2-quart pan and a heat-resistant bowl) or microwave, stirring frequently to combine.

6. Drizzle chocolate in striped pattern on top of coconut shreds.

7. Place in airtight container in refrigerator or freezer atop candy wrappers, parchment paper, or wax paper. Let sit at room temperature for about 20 minutes before serving.

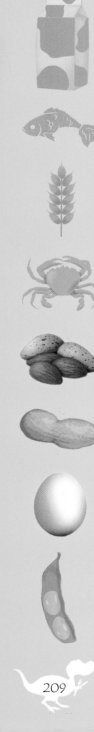

209

Special Treats

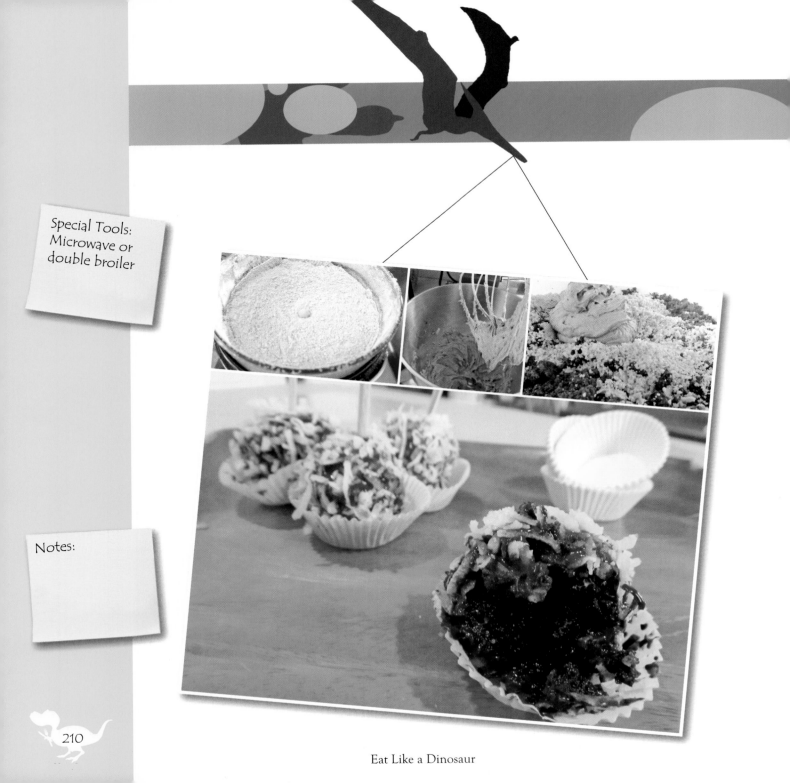

Notes:

210

Eat Like a Dinosaur

GERMAN CHOCOLATE CAKE BALLS

Makes 36 cake balls

German chocolate cake is flavored with nuts, caramel, coconut, and chocolate. It seemed a perfect choice, since that's all our favorite ingredients, to make our very first cake ball. If you've never had a cake ball before, they're awfully fun—like donut holes with frosting! It's a bit of work, but sure does impress.

INGREDIENTS

- ◇ 1 batch Red Brownie Cupcakes (p. 225)
- ◇ 1 batch Creamy Not Cheese Frosting (p. 227)
- ◇ 1 C walnuts, chopped
- ◇ 8 oz dark chocolate
- ◇ 2 Tbsp palm shortening or butter
- ◇ ½ C shredded unsweetened coconut

INSTRUCTIONS AND HOW KIDS CAN HELP

1. Crumble cooled cake into bowl.

2. Spoon frosting and walnuts over top of cake bits and mix by hand to incorporate.

3. Form into balls of cake and gently place on parchment or wax paper to set in refrigerator or freezer for at least 30 minutes to firm.

4. Melt chocolate with shortening in double boiler or microwave, stirring frequently to combine.

5. Coat each chilled cake ball in chocolate; set aside on parchment paper while finishing one dozen cake balls at a time, then roll in coconut—repeat for the next 2 dozen balls.

6. Return to refrigerator for another ten minutes to solidify chocolate before serving – store chilled for up to several days or in the freezer until ready to enjoy them.

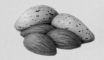
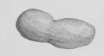

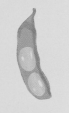

211

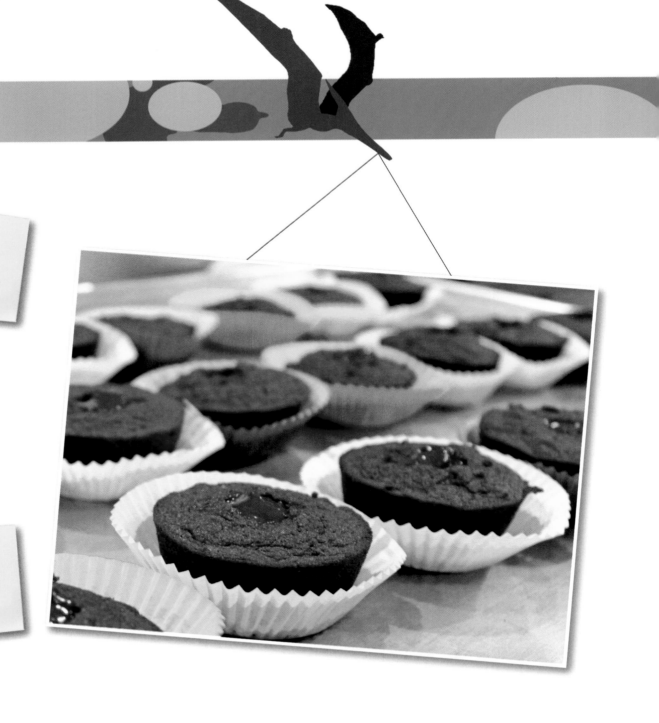

Notes:

Eat Like a Dinosaur

LAVA FUDGE CUPCAKES

Makes 18 cupcakes

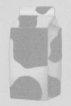

Lava is a super-hot substance that gurgles beneath the surface of Earth and sometimes erupts out of volcanoes. Lava can be anywhere from 1,300 to 2,200 degrees. It is made of rocks, dirt, and ash that are so hot they've melted together and become a fluid that flows along the ground burning up everything! After we learned about lava, we decided it'd be fun to make our own volcano cupcakes, with fudge "lava" inside.

INGREDIENTS

- ◇ 1 batch Red Brownie Cupcakes (p. 225), cooled
- ◇ 1 batch Fudge Sauce (p. 245), chilled
- ◇ 1 batch Chocolate Fudge Frosting (p. 215) or Creamy Not Cheese Frosting (p.227)
- ◇ ¼ cup chocolate chips (optional)

INSTRUCTIONS AND HOW KIDS CAN HELP

✋ Use an apple corer to remove the center of the thoroughly cooled cupcakes, careful not to punch through the liner.

✋ Use piping bag or squeeze bottle (save those empty mustard containers!) to fill the cored portion of the cupcake with Fudge Sauce, careful not to overflow.

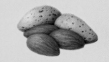

✋ Top with Chocolate Fudge Frosting or Creamy Not Cheese Frosting and sprinkle with mini chocolate chips for extra fun.

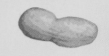

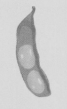

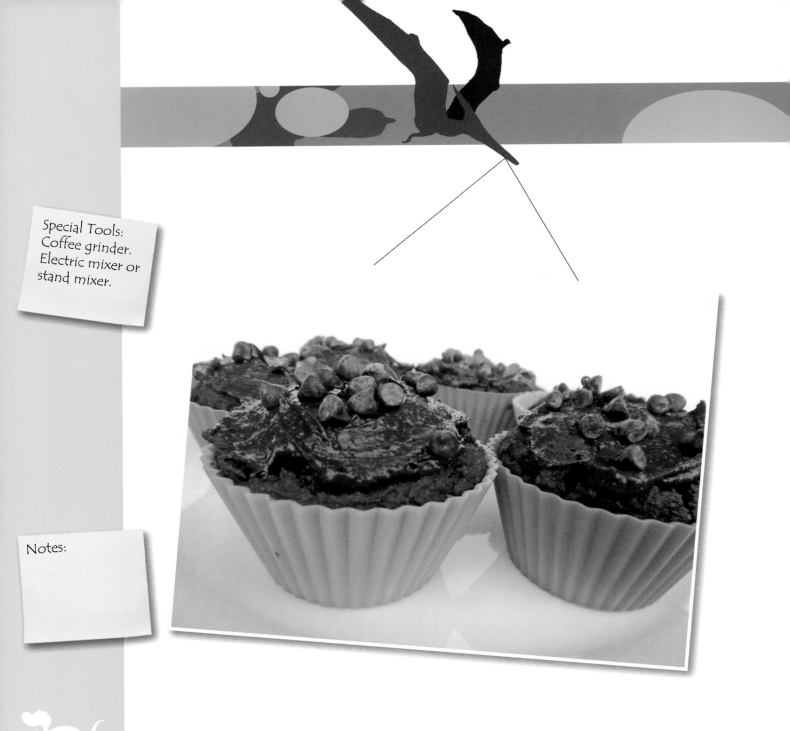

Special Tools:
Coffee grinder.
Electric mixer or
stand mixer.

Notes:

214

Eat Like a Dinosaur

CHOCOLATE FUDGE FROSTING

Ices 12 cupcakes

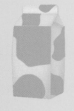
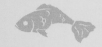

To make a chocolate sandwich, place this thick and fudgy frosting between two Chocolate Chip Cookies (p. 191). If you want a quadruple chocolate cupcake (that means four different kinds of chocolate), place this frosting on top of our Lava Fudge Cupcakes (p. 213) and then sprinkle with chocolate chips!

INGREDIENTS

- ◇ 1 C unrefined granulated sugar
- ◇ ½ C cocoa powder
- ◇ ¼ C palm shortening or butter
- ◇ 2 Tbsp unsweetened almond or hemp milk
- ◇ 1 Tbsp vanilla

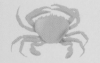
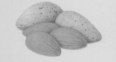
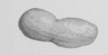

INSTRUCTIONS AND HOW KIDS CAN HELP

1. Use coffee grinder to powder sugar.

2. Mix all ingredients in an electric mixer until the consistency of icing, adding more cocoa powder if too runny or milk if frosting is too thick.

3. This gooey frosting pipes on very pretty with a swirl design, or simply spread onto cooled cupcakes.

4. Store chilled for up to several months.

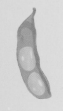

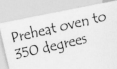

Preheat oven to 350 degrees

Special Tools:
Apple corer.
Piping bag or
squeeze bottle.

Notes:

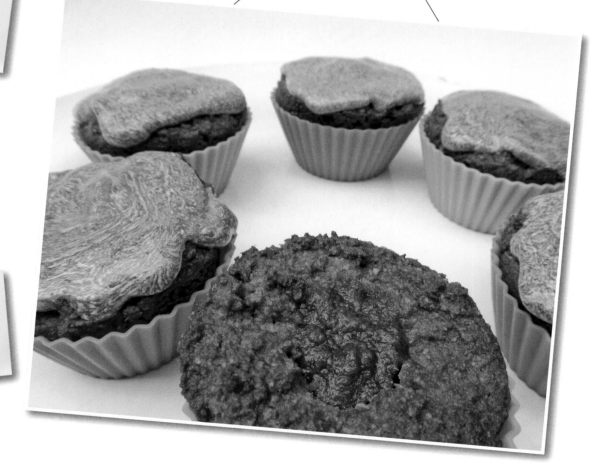

216

Apple Pie Cupcakes

Makes 12 cupcakes

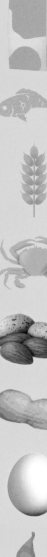

One of our favorite things to do on a rainy day is to watch food shows on TV. We especially love DC Cupcakes because that bakery is near to where we live! They punch a hole in the middle of their cupcakes and fill it with a delicious filling. What a great idea!

These cupcakes remind us of apple pie. We like to make them with our thick Applesauce (p. 131), but you can use any applesauce you have. If you use a store-bought brand, we suggest cooking it on the stovetop uncovered for a few minutes to thicken it, or it'll run out of the bottom of your cupcake!

INGREDIENTS

- 1½ C Applesauce (p. 131), separated
- ¼ C coconut oil, liquefied
- ¼ C honey
- 2 eggs
- 1 Tbsp vanilla

- 1½ C almond flour
- ½ C coconut flour
- 1½ tsp baking soda
- ¼ tsp salt

INSTRUCTIONS AND HOW KIDS CAN HELP

1. Beat together ½ cup applesauce with oil and honey.
2. Add eggs and vanilla while beating the wet mixture.
3. In a separate bowl, sift and combine the flours, baking soda, and salt.
4. Slowly add the dry ingredients to wet ingredients, while beating on low, until just combined.
5. Fill lined muffin cups ¾ full and bake at 350 degrees for 25 minutes, or until centers are firm.
6. Use an apple corer to remove the center of the thoroughly cooled cupcakes, careful not to punch through the liner.
7. Use piping bag or squeeze bottle (save those empty containers!) to fill the cored portion of the cupcake with thick applesauce, until just level with the cupcake.
8. Top with Caramel Icing (p. 219).
9. Store chilled for up to a week.

Special Treats

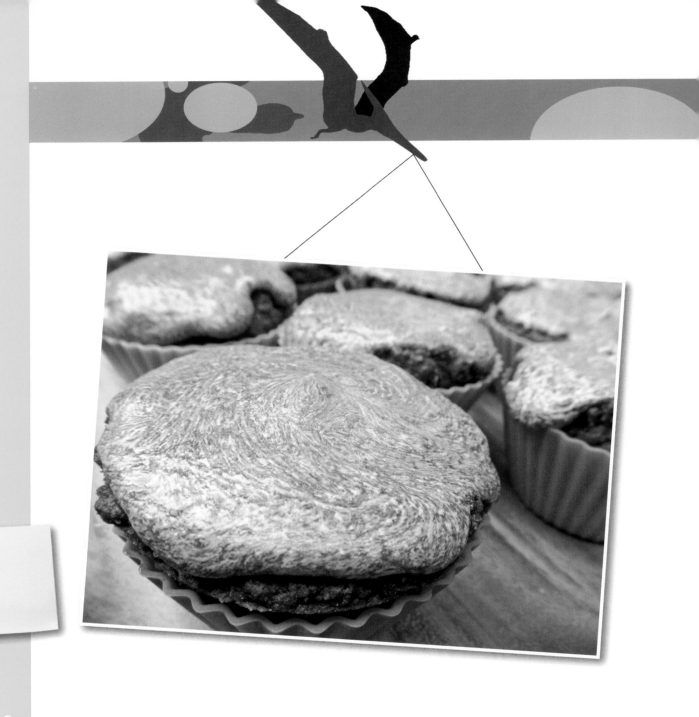

Eat Like a Dinosaur

Caramel Icing

Ices 12 cupcakes

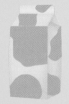

This icing is fun and quick to make, and it's really cool looking the way the sugar and icing swirl together. It'd be great on almost anything, but we recommend trying it with our Apple Pie Cupcakes (p. 217) and ZuCakes (p. 223)!

INGREDIENTS

- ❖ 1 C unrefined granulated sugar
- ❖ ¼ C palm shortening
- ❖ 1 Tbsp almond milk
- ❖ 1 tsp vanilla

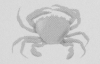
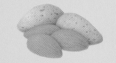
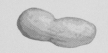

INSTRUCTIONS AND HOW KIDS CAN HELP

 Use coffee grinder to powder sugar.

Combine all ingredients in electric mixer, whip on high until icing is fluffy (add a

splash of almond milk or shortening if mixture is too dry or wet).

3. Store chilled for up to several months.

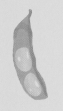

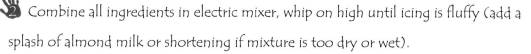

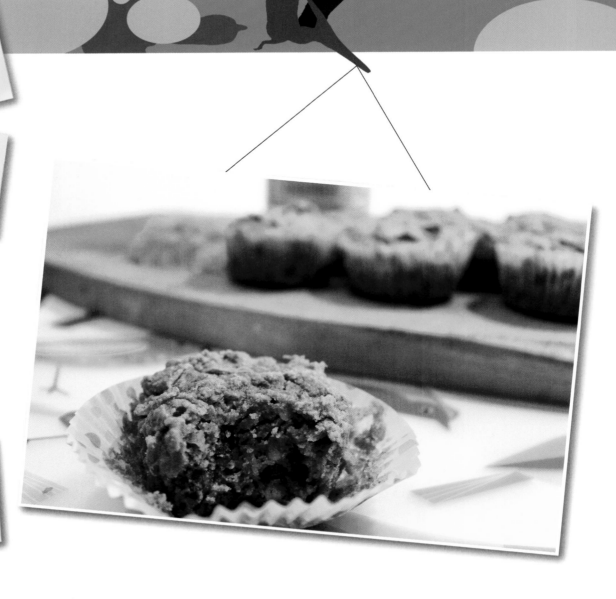

Preheat oven to 350 degree

Special Tools:
Electric mixer or stand mixer

Notes:

Eat Like a Dinosaur

GIGI'S CARROT CUPCAKES

Makes 1 dozen

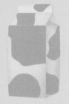

Stacy grew up loving carrot cake. Every birthday she'd ask for the same thing: her mom's (whom we call Gigi) carrot cake. What made it so amazingly delicious was the added crushed pineapple, which sweetened the cake and gave it great texture.

As a special surprise to Stacy, Matt came up with this recipe based on the flavors she grew up loving. The result is an amazingly moist and delicious muffin that is sweetened with only fruit. Healthy enough for any time of day, but rich enough for you to top with our Creamy Not Cheese Frosting (p. 227) for a delicious birthday treat.

INGREDIENTS

- 2 C almond flour
- 1 tsp baking soda
- ½ tsp salt
- ½ tsp nutmeg
- 1 Tbsp cinnamon
- ½ C dates, diced finely
- ½ C coconut oil, melted

- 2 eggs
- 1 Tbsp vanilla
- ½ C crushed pineapple, juice strained
- 1 C shredded carrots
- Optional: ½ C raisins
- Optional: ½ C walnuts, chopped

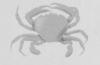

INSTRUCTIONS AND HOW KIDS CAN HELP

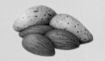

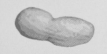

1. Mix together flour, soda, salt, nutmeg, and cinnamon.
2. In separate bowl cream together dates, oil, eggs, and vanilla using electric mixer or stand mixer.
3. Add dry ingredients to wet and mix until combined.
4. Fold in pineapple, carrots, raisins, and walnuts.
5. Distribute mixture into greased or lined muffin tin until ¾ full (about ¼ cup).
6. Bake at 350 degrees for 20-25 minutes for muffins.
7. Store chilled for a week or more.

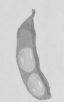

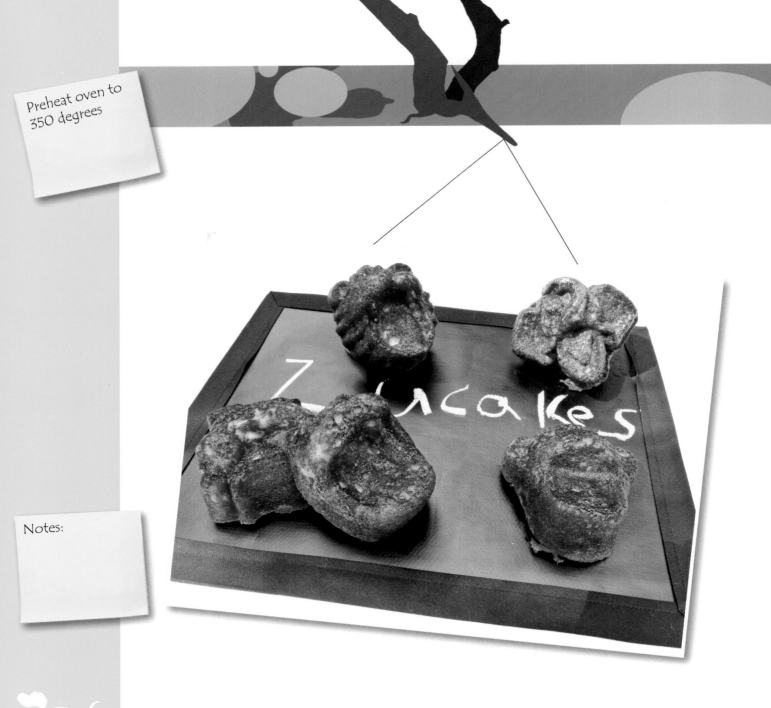

Notes:

Eat Like a Dinosaur

ZuCakes

12 medium cupcakes or 1 loaf

When we found a cake pan featuring zoo animals, the idea of a zucchini cake recipe called ZuCakes (pronounced zoo-cakes) became something we needed to invent. Zucchinis are naturally pretty sweet, and that means you don't need a lot of sugar.

The batter is pretty forgiving and would work as cupcakes, muffins, a loaf, or maybe even a birthday cake! This fun pan we used was perfect for scooping our Honey Nut Ice Cream (p. 237) in the animals' mouths, but we think our Creamy Not Cheese Frosting (p. 227) goes great with it too.

P.S. Save your drained pineapple juice to make our Pineapple, Mint, and Clementine Water (p. 187)!

INGREDIENTS

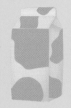

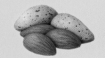
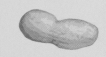

⋄ ½ C honey	⋄ 2 C almond flour
⋄ ¼ C coconut oil, liquefied	⋄ 1½ tsp baking soda
⋄ 3 eggs	⋄ ½ C zucchini, shredded
⋄ 1 Tbsp vanilla	⋄ 1 (18 oz) can crushed pineapple, juice drained

INSTRUCTIONS AND HOW KIDS CAN HELP

1. Mix together honey, coconut oil, eggs, and vanilla.
2. In a separate bowl, mix the flour and soda.
3. Beat the dry ingredients into the wet ingredients on low until incorporated.
4. Fold in zucchini and pineapple.
5. Grease your cake pans.
6. Fill your cupcake pans ¾ full.
7. Bake uncovered at 350 degrees for 30 minutes.
8. Store chilled for a week or more.

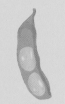

Preheat oven to 425 degrees, then turn down to 350 when beet is finished cooking.

Notes:

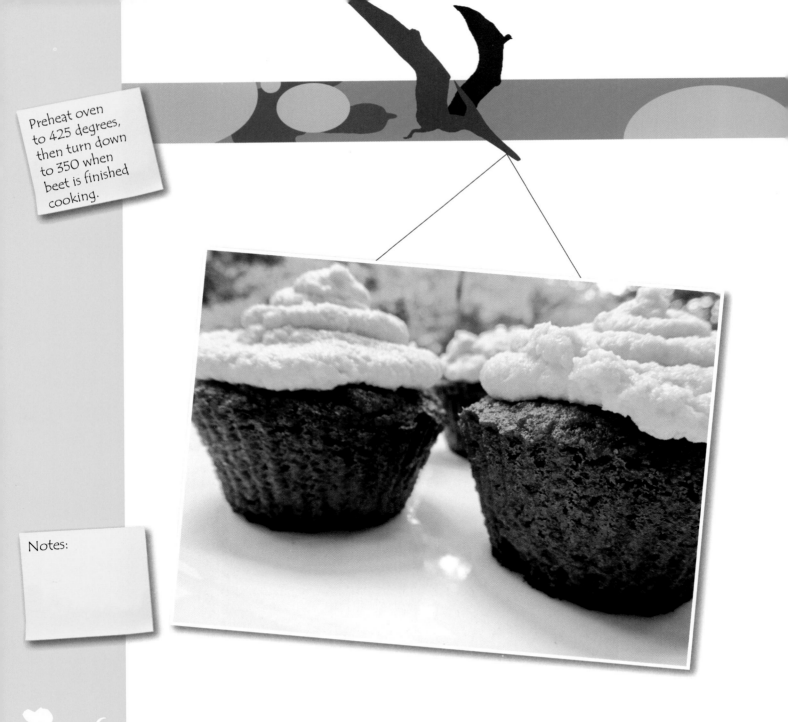

Eat Like a Dinosaur

RedBrownieCupcakes

Makes 18 cupcakes

One day it snowed nearly two whole feet at our house and we were completely stuck for two whole days. What were we going to do?

With a lot of time and a big idea to make cupcakes, we spent a few hours tasting recipes until we got this version of cupcakes just right. Usually these cupcakes are called red velvet, but we skip the food dye and use red beets instead to make them a little red. Next, we add a little extra chocolate to make them more like chocolate brownies.

We think this recipe is a lot of fun to make on a cold winter's day, but there's no reason you can't make it for a summer BBQ and put fresh berries on top.

You can also find this recipe in our Samoa Cake Balls (p. 209) and Lava Fudge Cupcakes (p. 213). We used the Creamy Not Cheese Frosting (p. 227) to decorate these in the pictures.

INGREDIENTS

- 1 medium red beet
- 1 Tbsp coconut oil
- 1 C fresh dates, (approximately 15)
- ½ C coconut oil
- ½ C palm shortening or butter
- ½ C unrefined granulated sugar
- ½ C full fat coconut milk
- 2 Tbsp vanilla extract
- 3 Tbsp apple cider vinegar
- ½ tsp lemon zest (half of one lemon)
- 8 eggs
- 1 C almond flour
- ½ C coconut flour
- 1/3 C cocoa powder
- 1 tsp baking powder
- 1 tsp baking soda
- 1 tsp sea salt

INSTRUCTIONS AND HOW KIDS CAN HELP

1. Wash, peel and dice beet. Coat evenly with coconut oil and roast for 20 minutes at 425 degrees until the texture is mushy like a banana.
2. If you are unable to find fresh dates, soften dehydrated dates by covering with boiling water for 15 minutes, then strain and purée with cooked beet and coconut milk.
3. Add to purée, oil, sugar, vanilla, vinegar, and zest until combined.
4. Transfer wet batter to bowl for electric mixer, add one egg at a time and beat in.
5. Sift together dry ingredients in a separate bowl.
6. Slowly add to wet ingredients as you beat until batter is formed.
7. Fill lined muffin cups ¾ full.
8. Bake at 350 degrees for 20 –30 minutes.
9. Store chilled for a week or more.

Special Treats

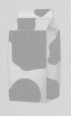

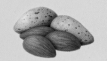
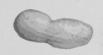

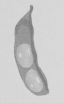

Special Tools:
Food processor
or blender

Notes:

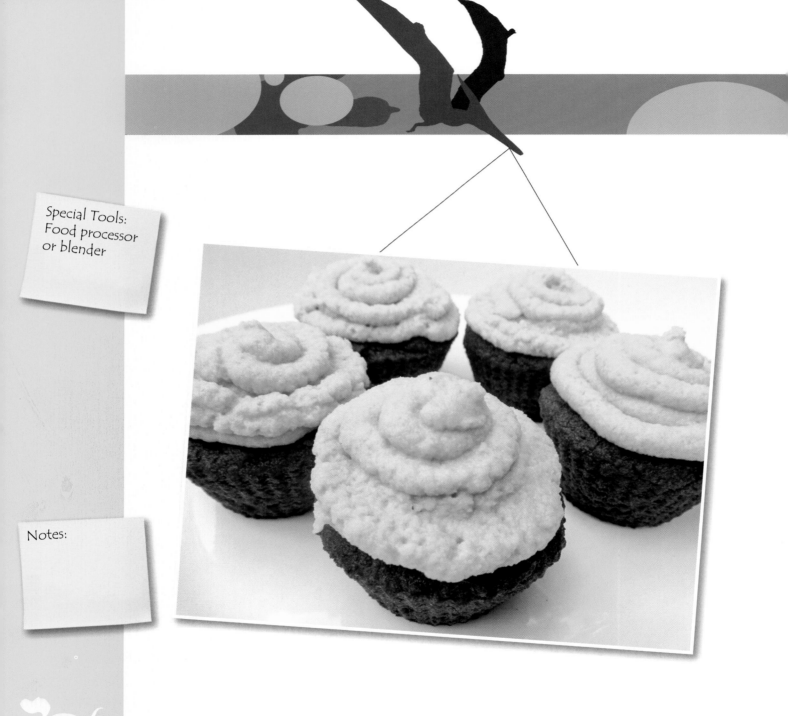

CREAMY NOT CHEESE FROSTING

Frosts 24 cupcakes

This creamy frosting has a long "waiting period" for preparation, but the results are worth the wait. It's pretty hard to make a plain frosting if you don't use milk, butter, or cream, but we think this recipe hits the bullseye. Try it on our Red Brownie Cupcakes (p. 225) or ZuCakes (p. 223) recipes!

INGREDIENTS

- 3 C raw macadamia nuts or raw cashews, soaked and rinsed (overnight, or at least 4 hours)
- ¼ C maple syrup
- ¼ C honey
- 1 Tbsp vanilla extract
- 1 Tbsp almond extract
- 1 Tbsp apple cider vinegar
- 2 tsp lemon juice

INSTRUCTIONS AND HOW KIDS CAN HELP

1. Combine all ingredients in a food processor or blender.
2. Scrape sides, making sure all pieces are puréed and incorporated.
3. If mixture does not yet resemble a frosting-like texture, pulse in 1 tablespoon almond milk (or any milk) a teaspoon at a time until rich and creamy.
4. Frost cupcakes to your liking. If using a piping bag ensure a wide tip to avoid nut pieces getting clogged.
5. Store chilled for up to several weeks.

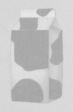

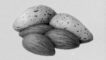
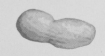

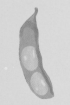

Notes:

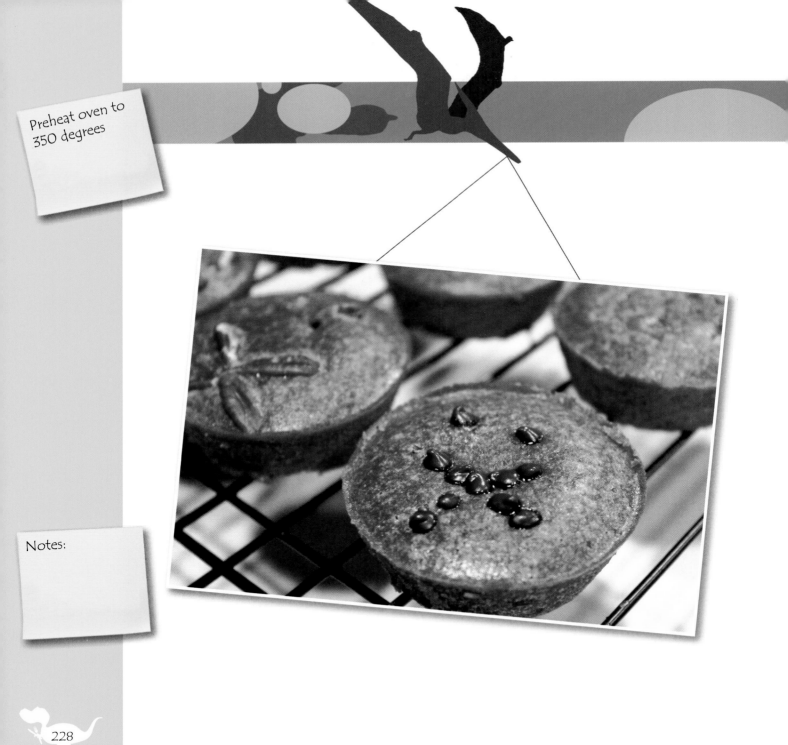

Eat Like a Dinosaur

Pumpkin Pucks

Makes 12 cupcakes

Matt used to love making pumpkin pies for Thanksgiving, but usually pumpkin pies are made with a canned, thick liquid made out of sugar and milk called sweetened condensed milk. That doesn't sound healthy at all! So we invented our own version of mini pumpkin pies, which we call pumpkin pucks! The inside is almost creamy and has plenty of pumpkin power in its punch!

INGREDIENTS

- 1 C pumpkin purée
- 1 C almond butter
- 1/4 C honey
- 2 Tbsp maple syrup
- 2 eggs
- 1/3 C almond flour
- 1 Tbsp cinnamon
- 1 tsp nutmeg
- 1/2 tsp salt
- 1/3 cup mini chocolate chips or chopped nuts for decorating (Optional)

INSTRUCTIONS AND HOW KIDS CAN HELP

1. With electric mixer or stand mixer, whip pumpkin and almond butter together until thoroughly combined.

2. Add honey and syrup and beat in eggs one at a time.

3. Add dry ingredients to wet and mix until just combined.

4. Fill muffin cups 3/4 full in greased muffin tin (they will not rise but more would be too dense).

5. Top with decorations if you choose, but we think they are perfect without anything.

6. Bake at 350 degrees for 20 minutes, will be firm to the touch but a testing knife or stick will not come out clean.

7. Store chilled for up to a week or me.

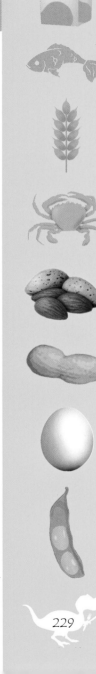

229

Special Treats

Special Tools:
Electric mixer.
Food processor.
Waffle iron,
preheated.

Notes:

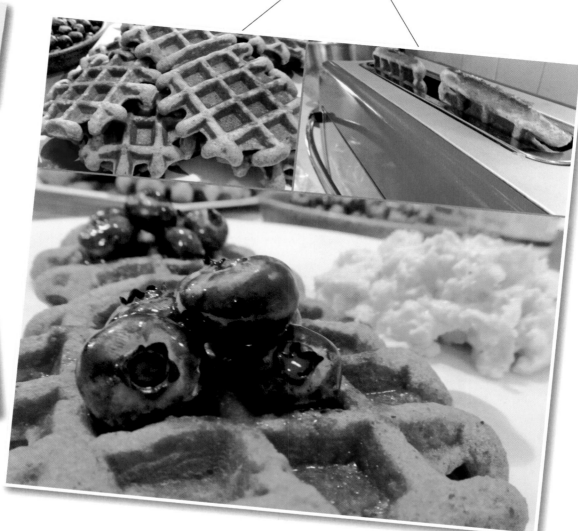

230

Eat Like a Dinosaur

FROZEN WAFFLES

Serves 6

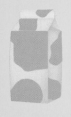

This happens to be one of our favorite recipes in the entire book. It has some surprising ingredients, but they come together so nicely that they really do taste and feel like the waffles you had before you ate like a dinosaur. Dinosaurs didn't have freezers or toaster ovens, but with this recipe you'll be able to have frozen waffles again, only without creating the extra trash from the box!

We like to make a double or triple batch of these and keep them stored in the freezer so that the boys can pop them in the toaster and make their own breakfast sometimes. They're great with all kinds of toppings—Cole loves them with apple butter and Finian insists on putting bacon and eggs on his and rolling it up like a taco. Wesley just loves eating them however we serve them!

INGREDIENTS

- ◇ 1 banana
- ◇ 1 apple, peeled and cored
- ◇ 1 C almond butter (or MaraNatha brand sunflower butter)
- ◇ 2 eggs

- ◇ 1 Tbsp arrowroot powder
- ◇ 1 Tbsp vanilla
- ◇ ½ tsp baking soda
- ◇ Oil for greasing waffle iron

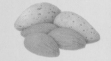

INSTRUCTIONS AND HOW KIDS CAN HELP

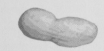

1. Purée apple and banana in food processor.
2. Use the whisk attachment on your electric mixer and whip almond butter on high for 2–3 minutes until smooth.
3. Add purée and remaining ingredients to whipped almond butter and continue to whip until combined.

4. Grease your hot waffle maker (for each waffle you make), we use Spectrum brand coconut oil spray.

5. Use about 1 ladle of batter per 8-by-4-inch waffle (do not fill up entire waffle maker, leave 40% unfilled, batter will spread) onto hot waffle iron for three to five minutes until browned, stiffened and cooked through. If your waffle is soft or floppy, it's not ready yet—keep cooking for another minute or two!

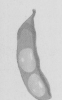

6. Eat immediately or store in freezer and make your own breakfast by reheating in the toaster.

Special Treats

Special Tools:
Food processor

Notes:

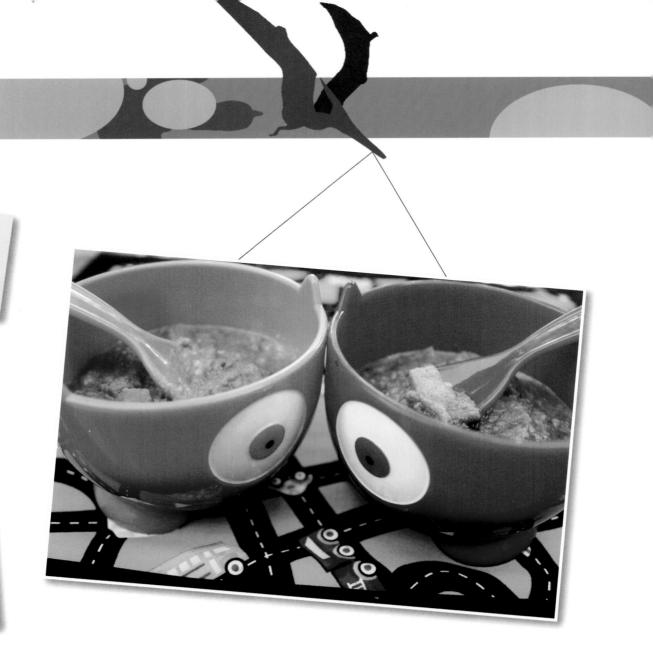

Eat Like a Dinosaur

CINNAMON APPLE CREAMED HOT CEREAL

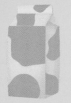

Serves 6-8

When I was growing up, my favorite breakfast was cream of wheat cereal. Cream of wheat was tiny bits of wheat cooked with milk. Now I realize that a dinosaur couldn't eat that! Still, sometimes you want to eat things even if it's not healthy for you.

Then one day as a birthday present, my boys made me this recipe and made me so happy! It tastes just like my cream of wheat breakfast, but only contains the healthy part! It was so good! Hope you love it, too!

INGREDIENTS

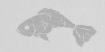

- ◇ 2 C raw walnuts
- ◇ 1 C raw macadamia nuts
- ◇ 1 C medjool dates, pitted and halved
- ◇ 2 apples, peeled and diced

- ◇ 1 Tbsp coconut oil
- ◇ 1 Tbsp ground cinnamon
- ◇ 2 C almond milk
- ◇ 1 14 oz can full fat coconut milk

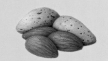

INSTRUCTIONS AND HOW KIDS CAN HELP

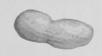

1. Combine nuts and dates in a food processor until ground into a fine meal, about 1 minute; set aside.

2. Sauté apples over medium heat in coconut oil until lightly browned, about 5 minutes.

3. Add nut and date mixture and cinnamon to apples and stir to incorporate, about 1 minute.

4. Reduce heat to low and add coconut and almond milk.

5. Stirring occasionally, let mixture cook uncovered until thickened, about 25 minutes.

6. Serve warm; store chilled in an airtight container for up to a week or two.

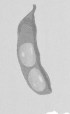

233

Special Tools:
Blender or food processor.
Ice Pop Molds.

Notes:

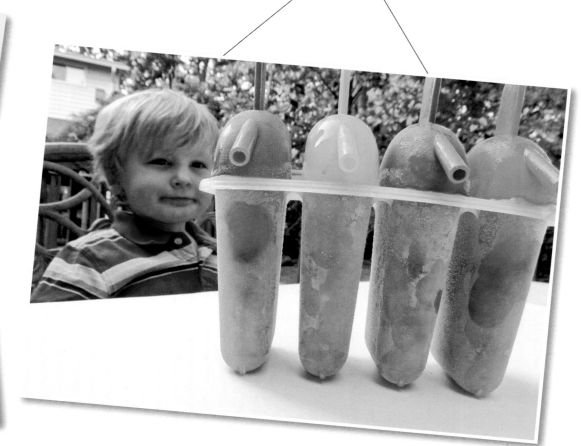

Eat Like a Dinosaur

WATERMELON ICE POPS

Makes 4

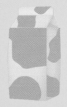

If you're like us, you probably have watermelon leftover after you've purchased a whole big melon. When it's been sitting in the refrigerator for a couple of days or so, the remaining pieces get really juicy—it's a perfect time to use them for making these ice pops.

We like to use Enjoy Life dairy-free, soy-free mini chocolate chips to make the ice pops look like they have watermelon seeds in them, but you can freeze them without the chocolate or add any chopped fruit you have available. It's a wonderful fruity and colorful base for whatever your imagination can think up!

INGREDIENTS

- ◇ 2 C very ripe and juicy watermelon
- ◇ ⅓ C mini chocolate chips

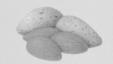

INSTRUCTIONS AND HOW KIDS CAN HELP

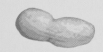

1. Remove any seeds and chop watermelon into 1- to 2-inch chunks.

2. Purée watermelon in a blender or food processor until very smooth.

3. Pour evenly into 4 ice pop molds, careful to not overfill.

4. Distribute chocolate chips by sprinkling on top of ice pop molds.

5. Gently stir in chocolate chips, ensuring they are distributed throughout popsicle. The chips should not sink to the bottom of the molds; the pulp of the watermelon will help them stay where they are "put" by being stirred.

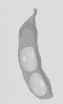

6. Freeze for several hours, until the ice pop is easily released by pulling on the stem (a quick dip in warm water will help).

Notes:

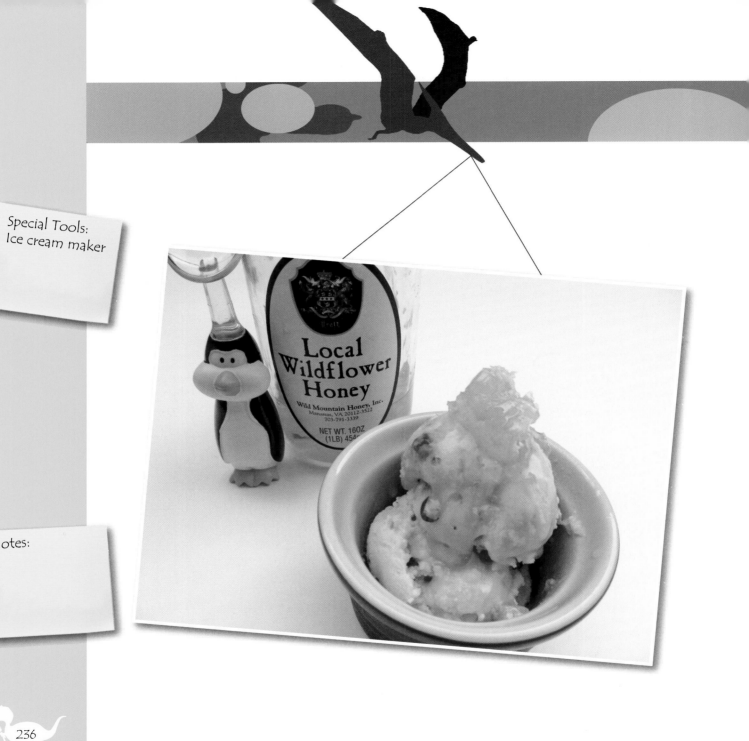

Eat Like a Dinosaur

HONEY NUT ICE CREAM

Makes a quart of ice cream

You might be missing your Honey Nut Cheerios, but this recipe will surely surpass any memory you had of those sugar bombs. Who'd have thought that ice cream was healthier than cereal?!

We like to use local wildflower honey we get at the farmers' market because it is rich and delicious. But the best part of using fresh local honey is that the pollen bees collect during the process of making honey helps your body handle the flower pollen in the air so that you sneeze less in the spring. Bees are super-awesome for the earth, too, and without them we might not have flowers or trees.

Next time your squeeze bear runs out, maybe you can get honey from a local bee keeper. You might even be able to find honeycomb, which makes a great topping for this ice cream! If you don't know what a honeycomb is, ask your parents to help you look it up—super-cool and interesting!

INGREDIENTS

- 1 (14 oz can) of full-fat coconut milk
- 2 C unsweetened almond or hemp milk
- ¼ C honey
- 1 Tbsp vanilla
- 1 C walnuts, chopped (use a food processor if you like a less chunky ice cream)
- Optional: honeycomb and drizzle of honey for topping

INSTRUCTIONS AND HOW KIDS CAN HELP

1. Whisk together the two milks until combined.
2. Add the honey and vanilla and whisk vigorously to combine.
3. Put this mixture in the ice cream maker and churn.
4. Allow your ice cream maker to churn for 20–30 minutes until thick and crystallized, adding walnuts halfway through.
5. Move to an airtight container and freeze ice cream after churning.

Best served after 1–4 hours after being frozen. If not eaten immediately, simply set the ice cream on the counter for 10-15 minutes prior to serving in order to soften.

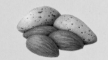
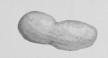

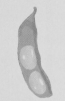

237

Special Tools:
Ice cream maker.
Strainer, colander
or cheesecloth.
Blender (optional).

Notes:

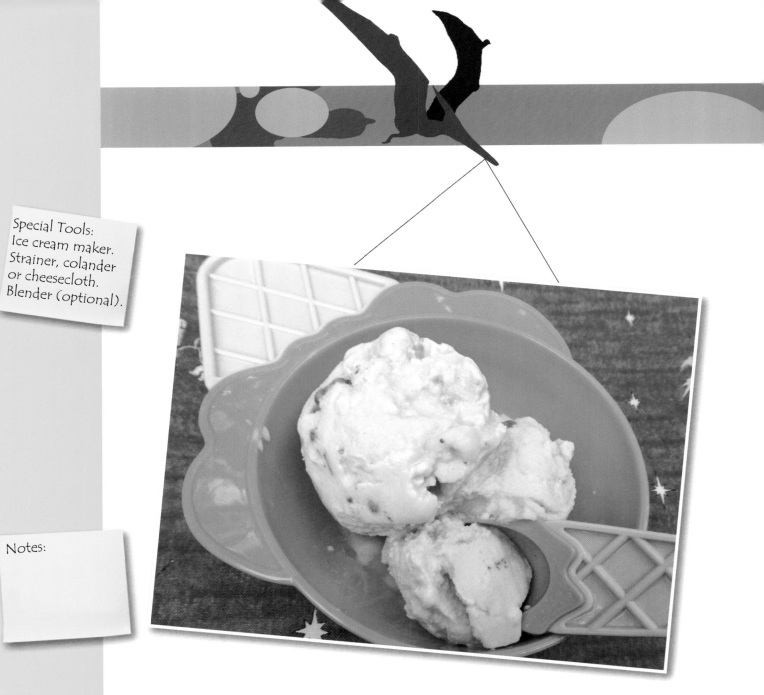

Eat Like a Dinosaur

Mint Chocolate Chip Ice Cream

Makes 1 quart

Before we started making mint ice cream ourselves, we called it "the green ice cream." Now we realize that the people who make green ice cream must be putting some scary stuff into it to make the color so bright, since ours isn't very green at all! Ours has just the same fresh taste we love, but without any additives. It's a surprising whitish color in the end, but our favorite green monsters love to eat it anyway because of its awesome flavor!

You might think you won't like this kind of ice cream, but it's our boys' favorite flavor by far. They love to go out to our garden (mint is the easiest thing to grow), then come in, fists full of mint, and request we make ice cream. Yum!

INGREDIENTS

- ◇ 2 C full-fat canned coconut milk
- ◇ 2 C unsweetened vanilla-flavor almond or hemp milk
- ◇ 1 C fresh mint leaves
- ◇ 1/3 C unrefined granulated sugar
- ◇ 1/2 C chocolate (use chips, minis, or even chunks: your choice!)

INSTRUCTIONS AND HOW KIDS CAN HELP

1. In medium sauce pan, combine milks, mint (whole leaves), and sugar and simmer over medium-low heat.

2. Simmer 15–20 minutes, letting little hands stir frequently until sugar is complete dissolved.

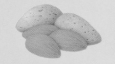

3. Strain out mint leaves, and place liquid in refrigerator to cool for at least 30 minutes. If you enjoy a strong mint flavor and want a vibrant bright green color, you could blend mixture until smooth instead of straining.

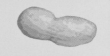

4. Churn cooled mixture in ice cream maker for 30 minutes, adding chocolate halfway through.

5. Transfer to airtight container and freeze ice cream after churning.

Best served 1–4 hours after being frozen. If not eaten immediately, simply set the ice cream on the counter for 10–15 minutes prior to serving in order to soften.

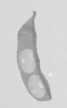

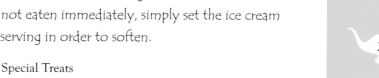

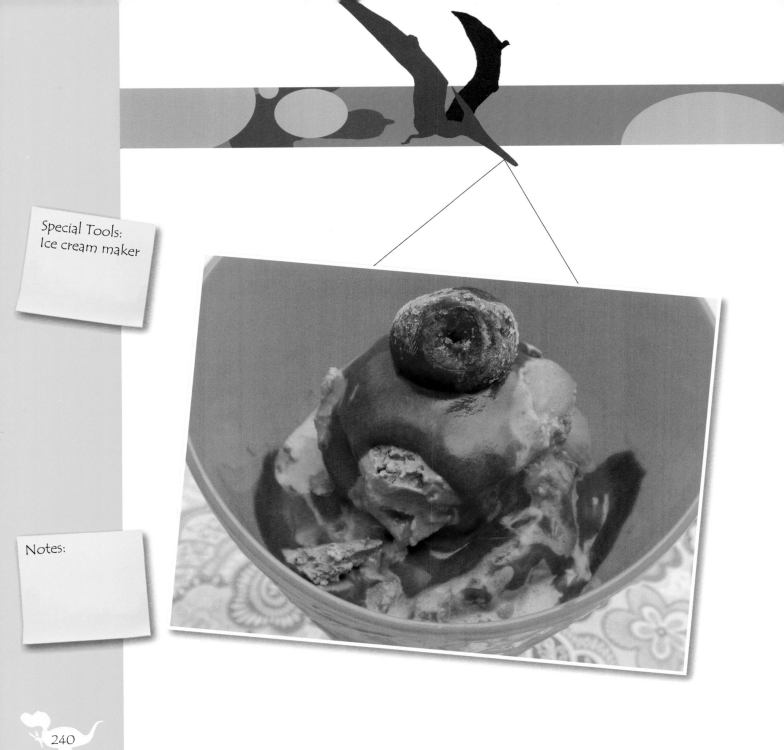

Eat Like a Dinosaur

CHOCOLATE NUT BUTTER RIPPLE ICE CREAM

Makes 1 quart

When Stacy was growing the boys in her belly, she'd make people drive as long as forty minutes one way to get her absolute favorite ice cream: peanut butter fudge. There was a particular restaurant that made it into a stupendous sundae. When she got the urge for that ice cream one summer after changing how we eat, we came up with this version instead. As you can see in the ingredients below, it includes sunflower seed butter, which works terrific. Instead of having to drive forty minutes one way these days, now all we have to do is make a quick trip to the panty and whip up our own ice cream.

INGREDIENTS

- 2 C full-fat canned coconut milk
- 2 C unsweetened vanilla-flavored almond or hemp milk
- ⅓ C unrefined granulated sugar
- ¼ C cocoa powder
- ½ C sunflower seed butter (we recommend SunButter or Trader Joe's brand)

INSTRUCTIONS AND HOW KIDS CAN HELP

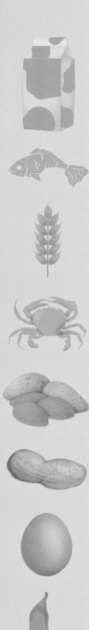

1. In medium sauce pan, combine milks, sugar, and cocoa powder and simmer over medium-low heat.

2. Simmer 10 minutes, letting little hands stir frequently until sugar and cocoa are complete dissolved.

3. Place in refrigerator to cool for at least 30 minutes.

4. Churn cooled mixture in ice cream maker for 30 minutes, until ice crystals have formed and mixture is very thick.

5. Transfer ice cream to an airtight storage container; slowly pour and fold the sunflower butter into the ice cream. Make sure to go slowly, only enough to evenly distribute the sunflower butter, but not incorporate it—or else you won't get a "ripple."

6. Freeze ice cream after churning.

Best served after 1–4 hours after being frozen. If not eaten immediately, simply set the ice cream on the counter for 10–15 minutes prior to serving in order to soften.

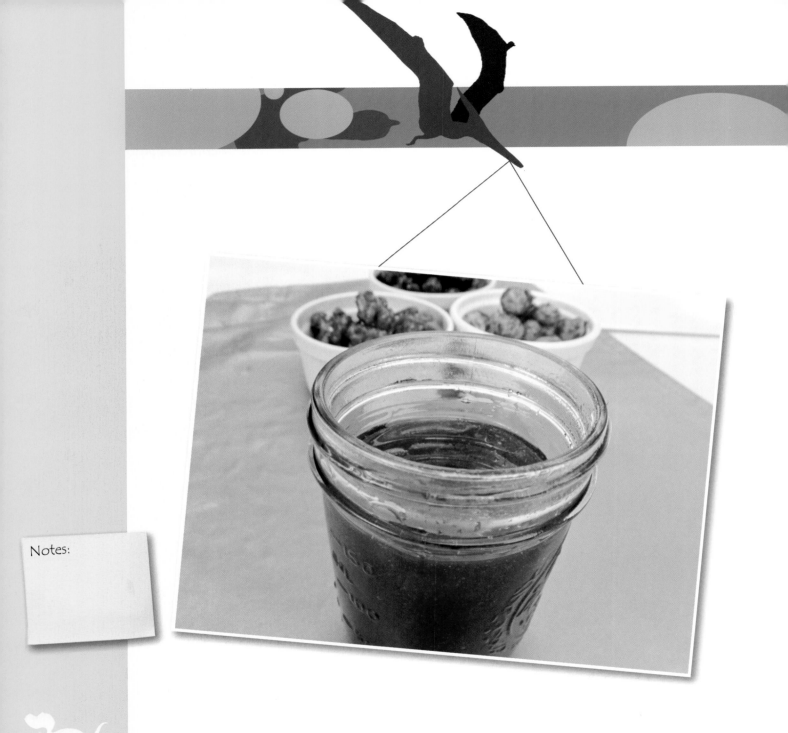

242

Eat Like a Dinosaur

CARAMEL SAUCE

Makes 1 cup

This versatile sauce is amazingly fun to make (science in action!) and useful on quite a few recipes. We use it to make Candied Nuts (p. 177), our Samoa Cake Balls (p. 209), and inside our homemade chocolate candies (see Make Your Own Candy, p. 267). It's delicious to drizzle it on special treats like ice cream.

Making caramel isn't as hard as it might seem, but it takes patience and lots and lots of stirring. Get your big muscle arm out and prepare to watch bubbles grow!

INGREDIENTS

- ½ C honey
- ½ C maple syrup
- ½ tsp baking soda

INSTRUCTIONS AND HOW KIDS CAN HELP

1. Warm large sauce pan over medium heat, add honey and maple syrup to warm pan—mixture should gently bubble, but if it begins to immediately boil and brown it has burned and you should start over.

2. Once gentle bubbles begin to form, turn heat to medium low; have little hands continuously stir (to prevent burning).

3. Mixture will bubble and potentially expand over edge of pot, if that happens, remove from heat and stir; return to heat once bubbles subside.

4. Once sauce has thickened and the color has darkened (about 10 minutes), remove from heat to add baking soda.

5. Whisk in baking soda thoroughly and continue to stir as it starts to expand and bubble; return to medium heat for 2–3 minutes. Whisk constantly until sauce has become a thick, rich, bubbly sauce that does not reduce when moved off of heat.

6. Remove from heat and let cool, stirring occasionally—sauce will reincorporate to a thick caramel consistency.

7. Serve and use warmed (heat in microwave or on stovetop).

8. Store in an airtight container for several months in refrigerator.

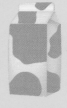

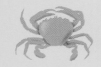
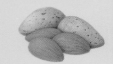
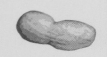

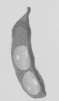

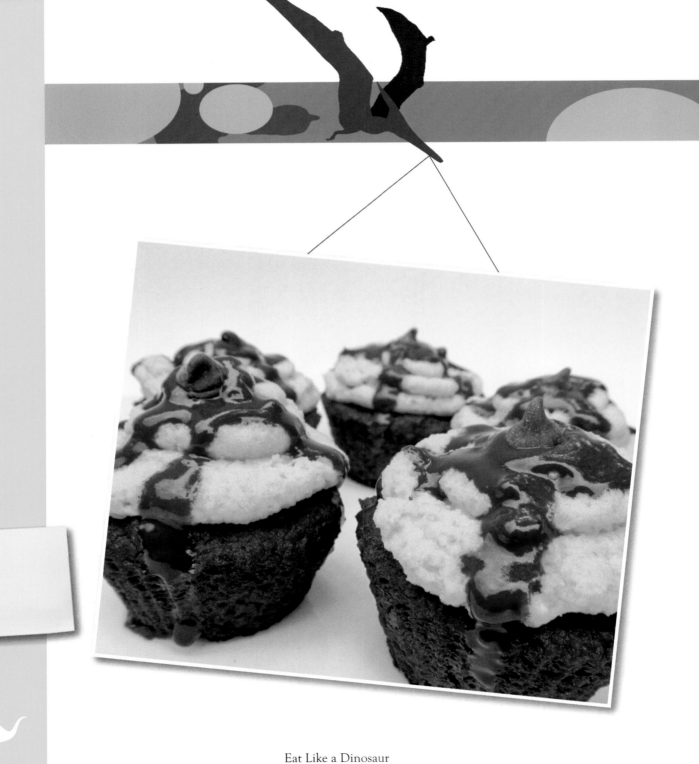

244

Eat Like a Dinosaur

FUDGE SAUCE

Makes 1½ cups

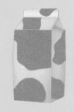

For a super-special treat, we like to use this as a fudge sauce for our Chocolate Nut Butter Ripple Ice Cream (p. 241) or as a filling in our Lava Fudge Cupcakes (p. 213). When this sauce is cold, its texture is thick like a pudding, which makes it great for dipping berries. When it's warm, it drizzles perfectly.

With this recipe it's fun to see how all the ingredients melt together and then become thick and oozy. We're sure you'll enjoy Fudge Sauce, but we must warn you that you'll probably need to wash your hands after you've eaten it. It always ends up all over our boys' faces!

INGREDIENTS

- ◇ ½ C unrefined granulated sugar
- ◇ ¼ C water
- ◇ ¼ C cocoa powder
- ◇ 1 tsp cinnamon
- ◇ ½ tsp salt

- ◇ ¾ C canned full-fat coconut milk
- ◇ 1 Tbsp arrowroot powder
- ◇ 4 Tbsp coconut oil
- ◇ 1 Tbsp vanilla extract

INSTRUCTIONS AND HOW KIDS CAN HELP

 Over low heat in a medium saucepan, stir together sugar, water, cocoa powder, cinnamon, and salt until incorporated, about 5 minutes.

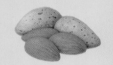 Pour in coconut milk and bring to a boil over medium heat, letting little hands stir constantly.

3. Once boiling, add arrowroot powder and boil gently for 3 minutes, stirring constantly (whip by hand as best you can).

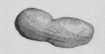 Once fully incorporated and lump free, reduce to simmer and stir occasionally over low heat for 20 minutes.

 Remove from heat and stir in vanilla and coconut oil.

6. Let cool at room temperature and store in airtight container in the refrigerator.

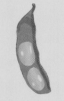

Special Treats

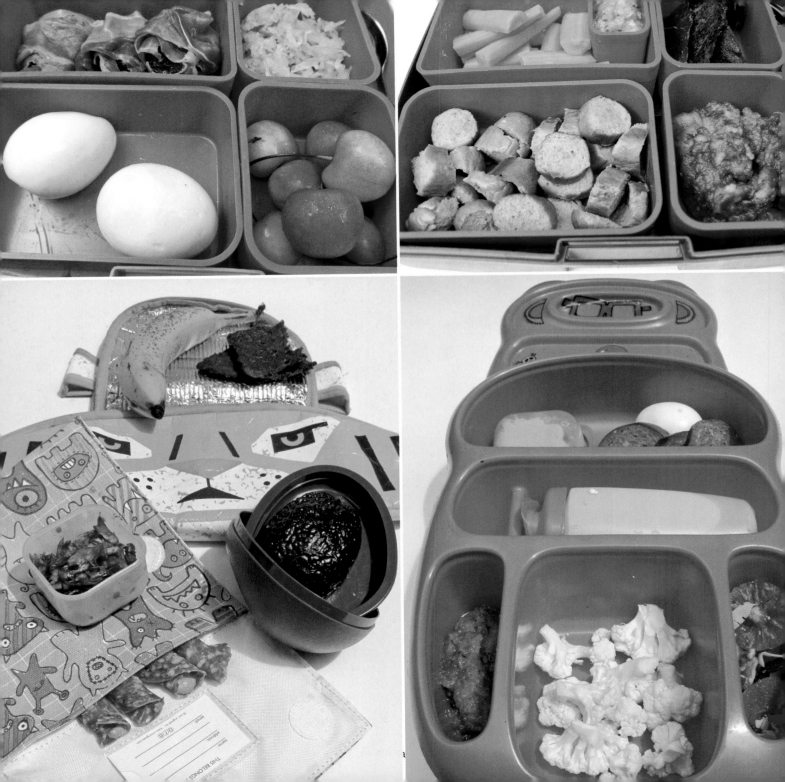

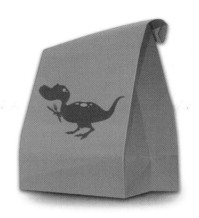

CHAPTER 8
PACKING LUNCHES

It's 8:15 AM. You've gotten everyone up, dressed, and fed, a series of events that we've all had some serious obstacles with. Now you have about two minutes and forty seconds to pack a lunch. So you reach for the sandwich bread... If you have kids in school, I'm sure you've gone through this exact scenario hundreds of times. We can relate because that's how it was for us, too.

The number one question we get from fellow parents who don't eat the same way as us is always: How do you pack lunches without bread? In fact, that's also the number one question we get from our diet allies. It seems that the sandwich paradigm is so ingrained that we are now unable to think of lunch without the bread-meat-cheese combination. And since most schools can't reheat a child's lunch, it seems almost impossible to fill the lunchbox with grain-free foods.

However, lunch really isn't as hard as you think it is. It took a few weeks (OK, maybe months) for us to finally reconceive what a packed lunch looks like, but now we've got it down. We realize there are actually more options without bread than there are with it. Once you throw away the sandwich crutch you'll find a whole world of possibilities.

The first and perhaps most effective way to rethink your lunch is to start by rethinking your lunchbox. Many of the healthy lunchbox examples we see online use images

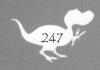

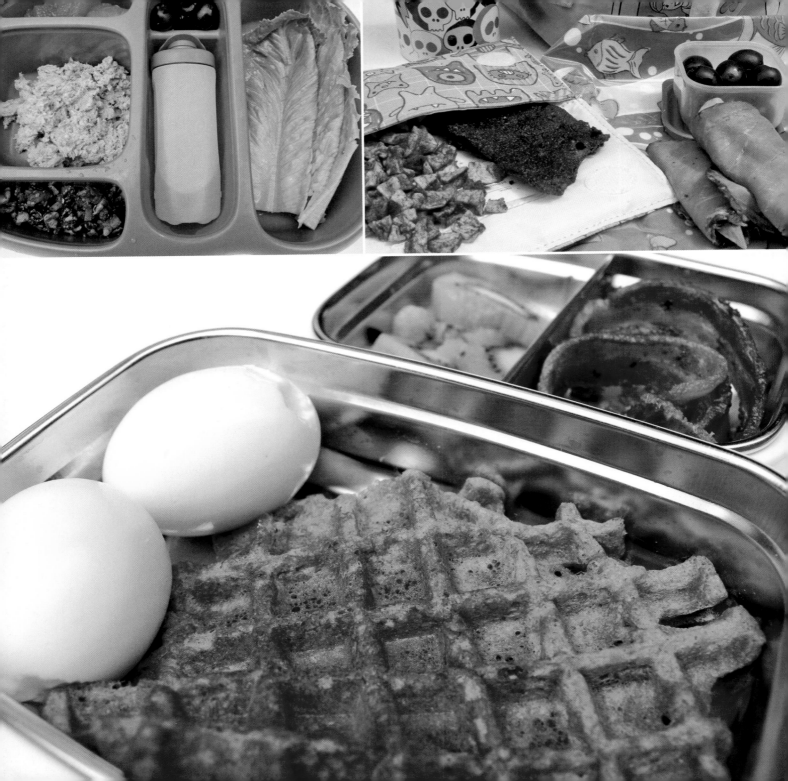

of individual glass containers. That's great, but our boys ought not to be trusted with breakable items at school! Instead, we often use container lunchboxes, as seen in our examples here, because they are convenient and store juicy items well without worries of breakage or leakage. The ones you see here are Bento brand Laptop Lunchbox Kits and Goodbyn. We like their larger version for our elementary school child and their smaller sized option for our preschoolers. They're BPA free and leak resistant (gotta put the lid on properly for it to be leak "proof"). These brands often come up at a discount at various websites and are well worth the investment.

Once you've gotten your container lunchbox, you need to fill the compartments with good, healthful foods. We still purchase lunchmeat as a quick and basic lunch food, but you should look for brands that only have meat and spices for ingredients. Avoid dextrose, sodium nitrite, and "natural flavors," which can be MSG. We like the Applegate Farms brand, which, while a little more expensive than others (their turkey bologna is the most affordable), never use the "Latin ingredients" that most brands do. We also get wonderful buffalo and venison salami from our butcher, farmers' market, and US Wellness Meats, our favorite online source. You can use your own roast chicken, roast beef, or pork belly slices to make (ahead of time) your own lunchmeat. Remember: if someone founded a company to make something, someone else first made it in their kitchen. And if it can be made in a kitchen, why not let that kitchen be yours?

We find that the key to success with packing lunches is playing to the kids' favorites. Our boys like lunchmeat, black olives, fruit, hard-boiled eggs, and avocado, so we figure out ways to always include at least one or two of these favorites in fun and interesting ways. In our case we try things like wrapping avocado wedges in roast beef or wrapping prosciutto around dates. Kids really like combining food into different combinations, and if one of those parts is already loved, you're halfway there. Would you believe that a favorite with our kids is pepperoni around a zucchini spear? Try new ideas because fun food is delicious food!

We have some seriously excited boys when we offer dip in their lunchboxes. You would not believe all the stuff we've gotten them to try simply by also providing a favorite sauce with it. Raw broccoli with pineapple sauce? Bratwurst with mustard? We've shared some of those sauces here in this book; in fact, we've devoted a whole section to them. Remember, to your kids a special sauce can be as simple as a mashed avocado.

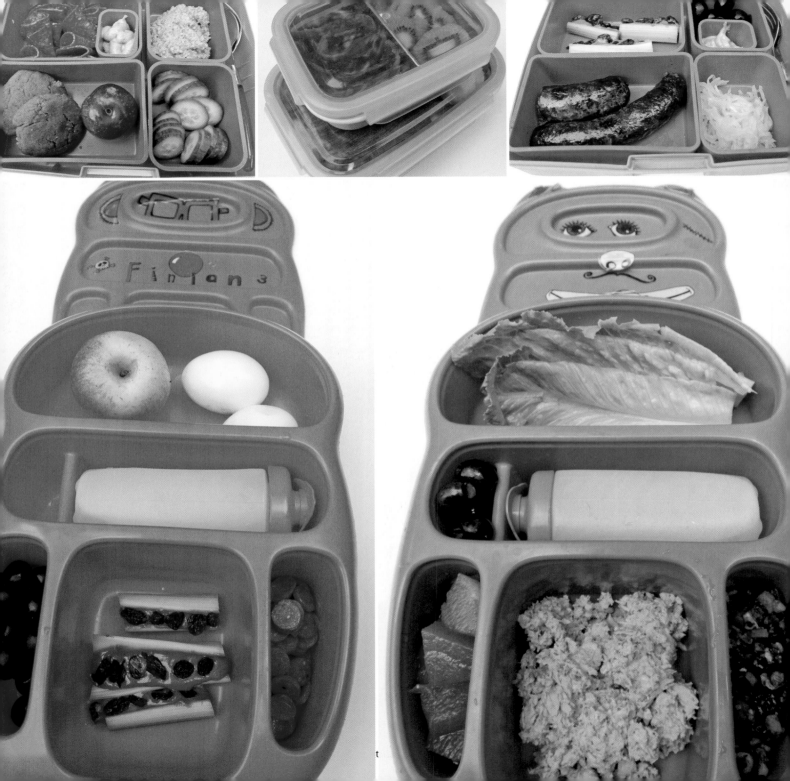

Tuna, salmon, egg, and chicken salads are very good for school lunches. We put them on lettuce, avocados, and celery sticks. Sometimes we use them as dip for carrots or apples. It's kind of a unique way to bring these things for lunch, but if your child loves it, they should have it. We were surprised when Cole asked for salmon salad on top of a green salad. And when he brought it to school, it impressed his classmates so much others started bringing it as well!

Leftovers from dinner can often be carried over to lunchtime, even if they can't be reheated. While I wouldn't send my children to school with curry, we'll place hamburgers or sausages or chicken legs in their lunches. Finn legendarily loves "Mock-a-mole hamburgers!" and doesn't mind them cold, so he brings that to school. If you're worried about the food keeping for the few hours before lunch, invest in some cheap ice packs to keep in their lunchbox. The Goodbyn brand has ice packs specifically designed for their boxes that we found for $2.50—a great investment!

While we try to avoid all processed foods, a few well-scouted box or bag foods will save you some time and make a good side dish. We've found dehydrated fruits and vegetables work really well, homemade or otherwise. And let your children pick out their own trail mix using their favorite nuts and dried fruit. We keep a big bag in the pantry and dole it out as the days go by.

And remember, kids have days where they just go, go, go, so always pack more than you think they could ever possibly eat! Otherwise, they might come home and say they were hungry for a snack so the teacher gave them Goldfish, Ritz, or Oreos.

Whatever lunch you pack or packing device you use, just make it fun and exciting for the kids. Write notes to surprise them, and make sure to pack one item they will be super excited to find. It's hard to be different, but if the other children see that your child's food is colorful and exciting, and they always have something cool like dips or wrapped food, then the other kids will be curious (read: jealous) instead of mean about your child's difference. And your child will feel proud of his or her lunch.

Eating healthy doesn't always have to be about getting out a book and looking up a recipe. Sometimes food can be about learning to do things yourself. In this section, you can get some cool ideas for different ways to have a fun time while learning about food with "little hands" helping.

These are some of our favorite things to do together as a family when we have a little more time than usual. Weekends are great for cooking together in the kitchen, experimenting with recipes, and shopping for kitchen gadgets and toys. If your family has time on the weekend, or if they ask what you'd like to do, these are some great ways to spend time together and learn at the same time!

And of course, the best thing about doing projects with food is that at the end of the project, you get to eat!

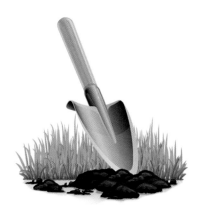

CHAPTER 9
PROJECTS

HOT POT

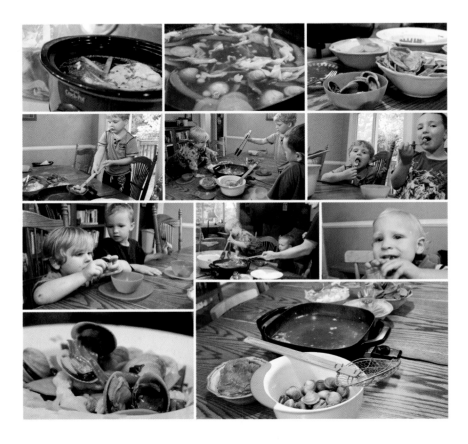

We love to explore new kinds of foods and were excited to find a new way to eat Asian cuisine: hot pot! Hot pot is a flavorful stock brought to a boil (bubbles in the water from heat) that you plop meat and vegetables into for cooking at your table! We loved eating at a local hot pot restaurant so much that we learned how to make it on our own.

We go to the Asian market and pick out which ingredients we want to try, come home, get everything prepared, and then poach away in some delicious and nutritious Bone Stock (p. 133). It's so easy to do, too!

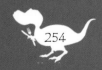

Eat Like a Dinosaur

STEP ONE: Figure out your heating device. You'll need an electric wok or fondue pot.

STEP TWO: Prepare your meats and veggies. Here are some things we love to cook in our hot pot:

- Shrimp
- Squid
- Scallops
- Mussels
- Clams
- Thinly sliced beef brisket
- Par-boiled quail eggs (let them finish cooking in the poaching liquid)
- Evenly sized vegetable pieces like carrots, snow peas, sugar snap peas, okra
- Greens like sliced cabbage, spinach, or kale

STEP THREE: Get your stock ready. Heat two quarts of Bone Stock (p. 133) to boiling (we suggest the stovetop first and then transfer to the tabletop device to maintain a boil). Add flavorings of your choice. We like 1 teaspoon of grated ginger, 1 tablespoon of fish sauce, 1 tablespoon of coconut aminos, and 2 sliced green onions. Then it's fun time! Drop in your food and cook it up!

STEP FOUR: Use tongs, a spider, or slotted spoons to drop foods into the poaching broth. Cook meat until light pink or brown, cook vegetables to your liking. For mussels and clams, once their shells open, cook for 1 minute longer. Remove all items from the poaching liquid once cooked and try to build a pile for everyone to get some. Once cooked you could even dip the food into little dipping dishes filled with coconut aminos, fish sauce, tamari, or sriracha.

MAKE YOUR OWN NIGHT:
KABOBS, TACOS, OMELETS

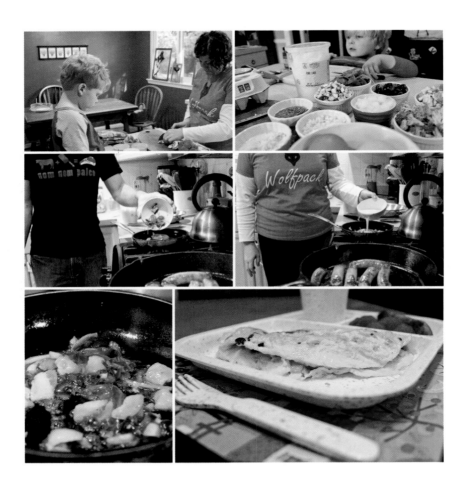

Some nights we get home and all we want is something a little different for dinner. That's when we have a "Make Your Own" night. It's a great way for the whole family to have fun in the kitchen together. There are many ways to do it, none wrong. We like to do omelet nights, kabob nights, and taco nights.

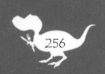

We've noticed that a lot of kids like "Breakfast for dinner!" For us, that used to be pancakes with sugary syrup, muffins, and toast. But that's not enough real food for a dinosaur! It's much more filling and fun to beat a dozen eggs, then let each person scoop eggs into the pan and sprinkle on their own fillings. Let it cook, fold it up, and you're ready for dinner!

HERE'S OUR FAVORITE FILLINGS:

- Black olives

- Ham cubes

- Bacon

- Salami

- Broccoli

- Avocado

- Diced tomatoes

- Diced squash

- Sautéed onions

- Sautéed mushrooms

- Sautéed peppers

- Herbs (oregano, basil, and thyme)

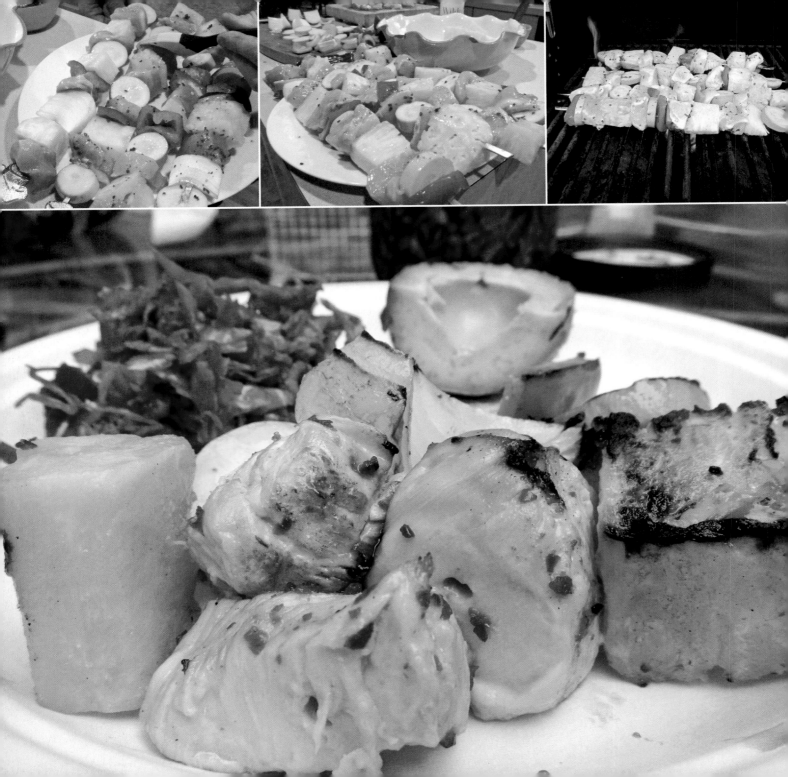

Kabobs are made by putting meat and vegetables on a big stick, and then placing the stick onto the grill. When we prepare them, we feel like pirates swording our veggies or knights jousting our dinner! Anything that can be cut into a large dice or is already round can be skewered on a stick. Remember to marinade your meat ahead of time because it will make it even better—use the marinades from our jerkys if you need inspiration.

Note: Make sure to soak wooden sticks in water for an hour before you cook them so they don't catch on fire!

SOME OF OUR FAVORITES ARE:

- Bacon-wrapped scallops
- Chicken
- Steak
- Shrimp
- Sweet bell peppers
- Cherry tomatoes
- Pineapple
- Zucchini
- Yellow squash
- Onion wedges

When we're in the mood for a fiesta, nothing is more satisfying than holding a make-your-own tacos and fajitas night. Wait, you say, what do you do about tortillas? Oh, that's simple: we use lettuce leaves! You'll be surprised how fun and crispy your taco will be. If you don't like lettuce, just make a big pile on your plate and dig in with a fork! To prepare, simply create a seasoning mix for your meat using chili powder, garlic, and cumin, then prepare these toppings:

- Ground meat (beef, venison, turkey, bison, you name it!)
- Sliced flank steak
- Grilled chicken (breast or thigh)
- Sliced sweet bell peppers
- Caramelized onions (sauté your onions with your meat and they become sweet)
- Diced tomatoes
- Guacamole (or sliced avocados)
- Salsa verde (sweet, mild green salsa)
- Red salsa

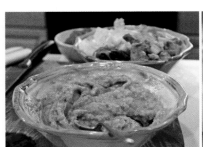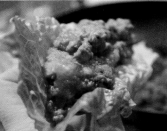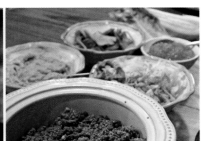

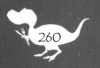

MAKE YOUR OWN
FRUIT & NUT BARS

When you go into a grocery store you can usually find a huge shelf full of all kinds of protein bars, power bars, fruit bars, and granola bars. Almost all of these could be re-named "SUGAR BAR" because they are made with ingredients that can make us sick. Fortunately, there are a few healthy bars out there. They are usually made exclusively from dried fruit (usually dates) and chopped nuts. Although these bars are delicious and much healthier than their grocery store neighbors, they too can contain a lot of sugar and be very expensive.

We suggest that you get the fruits and nuts you love and make your own bars. Why bother buying a bar when you can make the exact flavor you love at home! We always say that if you know the ingredients, you can make it. So we did, and boy are we glad!

The process for making these bars is (promise you can keep our super secret?) EASY! You need a food processor, but we almost always see one at our local thrift store for less than $10, so hopefully you can find a cheap one if you don't already have one.

STEP ONE: Figure out what ingredients you like and put them all together. Chop the entire mixture up in the food processor.

STEP TWO: Form a dough by rolling it into a ball and then simply place the dough between two sheets of wax paper or plastic and roll it flat (we like a thin bar so that it is a seemingly bigger portion but not a huge sugar load).

STEP THREE: Cut it into bars and store them in airtight containers. They last at room temperature for several days, and they last for up to several months in the refrigerator. We like to put them in a diaper bag, book bag, or a purse for when our tummies are rumbling and we're stranded without other paleo options.

FRUIT AND NUT BAR RECIPES

Below are some combinations that we like. The trick is that whatever amount of fruit you have, you have the same amount of nuts or less. We find that using fresh Medjool dates offers the best consistency, but dried dates are more shelf stable and do not need to be refrigerated. Try out whichever you prefer, and make sure to play with your favorite fruits and nuts.

Sugar Cookie Bar

These bars are Daddy's favorite. Bars that contain the same ingredients claim they taste like cashew cookies, but we think they taste like sugar cookies because they're so sweet and delicious.

> 1 C dates
> 1 C cashews

Movie Bars

We call these Movie Bars because we like to save them for special treats, like going to the movies. The chocolate chips add something super-special.

> 1 C dates
> ¼ C coconut flakes
> ¼ C dark chocolate chips
> 1 C macadamia nuts

Winter Rainbow Bar

Cole loves these bars because their flavors and colors remind him of Christmas. Pistachios are a fun green nut you may not have tried, but Hulk thinks you should!

½ C dates

½ C cranberries

1 C pistachio nuts

Papi's Bars

Grandpa sometimes needs a little help loving our foods, so we made this flavor for him using his two favorites: almonds and apricots. Since we almost always have these ingredients in the house, this is our go-to flavor.

½ C dates

½ C dried apricots

1 C almonds

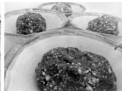
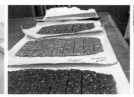

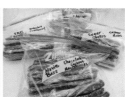

TRAIL MIX

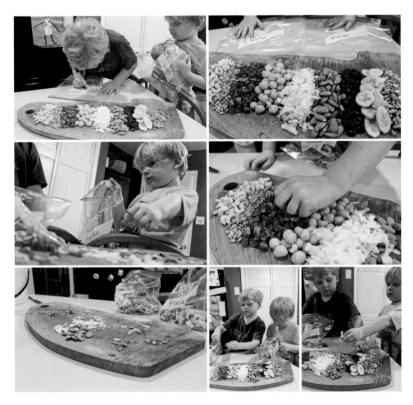

Another take-along snack we love to make is "trail mix." Many trail mixes claim to give you energy on the go, but they include chocolate candies, which does not give you healthy energy. But trail mix can be healthy when you make it on your own.

The boys love it when we call them in to "make your own trail mix for the week." We keep our pantry full of a lot of the ingredients, and our boys get to choose what they want in their trail mix. They fill up a bag or container that they know is just for them, and then we store the bags and containers in an accessible place for when their tummies are rumbling.

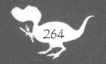

Eat Like a Dinosaur

BELOW IS A LIST OF OUR FAVORITE INGREDIENTS. JUST MAKE SURE TO CHOOSE UNSWEETENED AND UNSULFURED WHEN YOU'RE ABLE.

- Sunflower seeds
- Cinnamon Apple Tidbits (p. 167)
- Macadamia nuts
- Coconut flakes
- Almonds
- Dried cranberries
- Banana chips
- Pistachios
- Walnuts
- Cashews
- Apple Rings (p. 165)
- Dried apricots
- Dried cherries
- Pineapple (chips or dried)
- Chopped dry dates
- Raisins

We're not big fans of dried mango or blueberries because they can get sticky in the bag. But with all of the choices above, as well as others not listed, your child will truly feel their snack is custom made. And adults will be thrilled they don't have to do a thing!

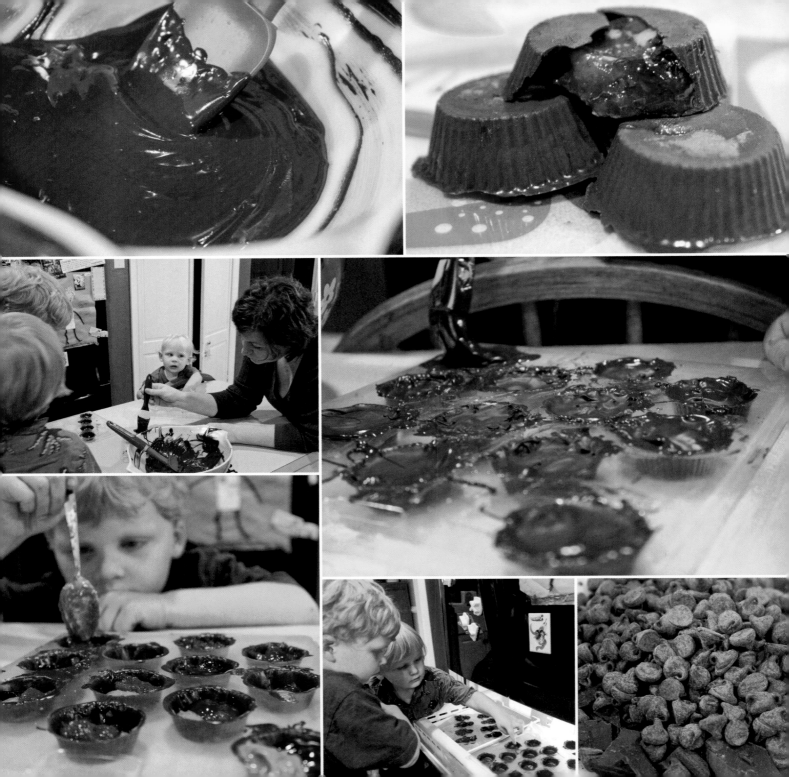

MAKE YOUR OWN CANDY

When the holidays come around, we like to give our friends and family candy for gifts and party favors. It sounds very difficult, but it's really not. All you need is some dark chocolate, some candy molds, and some imagination. We got our first mold years ago on a whim and have created thousands of candies since then. We hope we inspire you to try this yourself and figure out your own favorite treat.

STEP ONE: First, get a mold for your candies. The simpler and deeper the mold the easier it will be for you. You'll be tempted to purchase the fancy character molds, but the simple peanut butter cup is our favorite because it's the easiest. They are surprisingly cheap and easy to find at craft stores or online (about two dollars for a 12-candy tray).

STEP TWO: Melt 8 ounces of dark chocolate in a double boiler (we make our own with a 2-quart pan and a heat-resistant bowl) with two tablespoons of palm shortening or butter.

STEP THREE: Use a small spoon or pastry brush and paint the inside of the candy mold. This is the most fun part for kids! Our boys spend a painstakingly long time painting each individual cup, making sure that the mold is entirely covered and no holes remain (or your filling will ooze out).

STEP FOUR: Freeze it for a few minutes to harden. Make the fillings while you wait.

STEP FIVE: Then take out the mold and fill it about ¾ full with filling.

STEP SIX: Return to freezer for at least half an hour for the center to harden. Then finish painting the mold with a thick layer so that the chocolate is sealed. Freeze for a final half hour and you've got candy!

Chocolate Candy Recipes

Coconut Candy: On the stovetop combine $2/3$ cups shredded coconut, 2 tablespoons coconut cream, 2 tablespoons palm shortening, and 2 tablespoons maple syrup. Cook it on low until a paste is formed. Add this to the middle of the chocolate. If you really want to make it taste like the famous candy, add an almond.

Nut Butter Jelly Time! We like to pull out our favorite juice-sweetened jelly—often cherry, strawberry, or apple butter—and almond butter or sunflower butter and make a "PBJ" candy. Simply spoon a little of each into the candy for a classic combination. Just don't overfill!

For a Caramel Candy, place a walnut at the bottom of the candy and use our Caramel Sauce (p. 243) to fill the rest.

The best thing about candies? They can stay in your freezer for a long time and be eaten when you have surprise guests who are looking for a bite of chocolate. And really, with candy molds it's a simple process to do. Nothing sticking to pans, nothing to grease or bake. Just pop them out and serve!

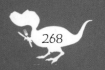

FARMERS' MARKET

Every Saturday morning (except in the winter), we get up early, eat breakfast, and drive or walk to our local farmers' market. In most every suburban and urban area in the United States you will find open-air markets where local growers gather to sell to YOU. We think the farmers' market is the most exciting place you can visit in your neighborhood.

Take the time to look up when and where your local market assembles and make it a weekly appointment to go there. If you have several, visit each one and figure out which one is your favorite. There are usually different types of vendors at each. During the spring and summer, we try to make it our main source to get fruits and vegetables. During the winter we are sad it's not open, but we are also happy that the farmers get a break and can spend time with their families.

There are many advantages to shopping the market. For one, you can be sure the produce is fresh because they usually pick it the day before. You will often have access to one of the growers in person, so you can ask about growing conditions, ask for recommendations, and ask for bulk discounts on overripe tomatoes that you might want to use for Ketchup (p. 143), or peaches or dried apples for Fruit Leather Roll-Ups (p. 169). You will also know that everything you get locally is in season and not shipped in from a different climate or grown chemically. Plus, the variety is fantastic.

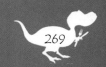

269

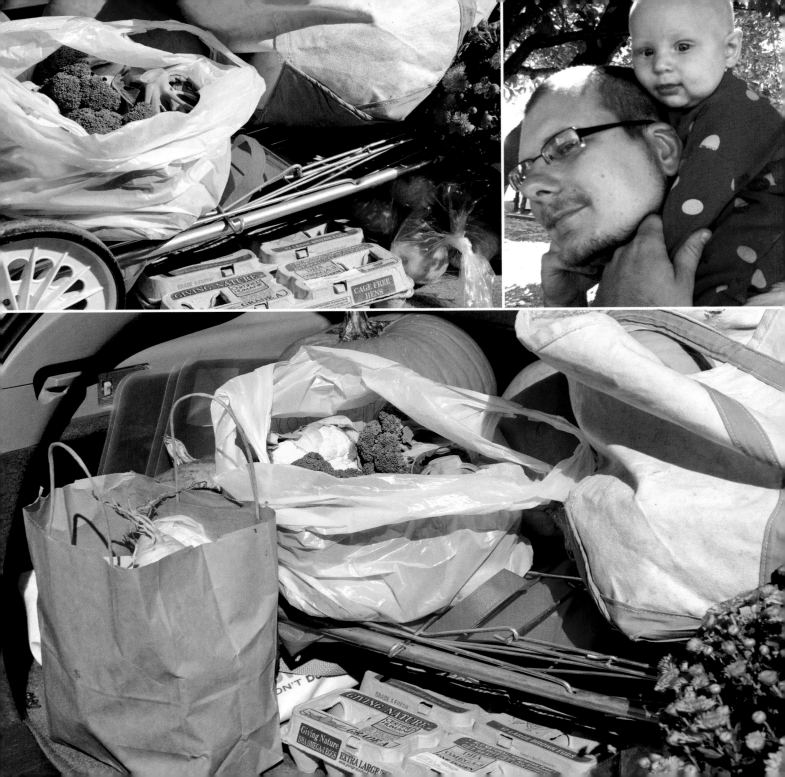

HERE ARE A FEW TIPS TO SUCCEED AND MAKE YOU FEEL MORE COMFORTABLE ABOUT WHAT YOU'RE BUYING:

~ Ask the vendor where their food is grown. Sometimes nonlocal vendors are simply selling grocery store quality produce under a tent, but hopefully that's not likely.

~ Ask if the vendor is certified organic; but don't be afraid if they're not. Organic pesticides can be problematic too, and the "organic" certification is costly. Most family farms are pesticide-free, using natural irrigation practices, and are happy to talk about their techniques instead of just wearing an "organic" sticker.

~ Get to know the farmers! Ask them their names, introduce yourself, bring your kids and let them ask questions about farming and what they recommend. Let your kids pay for the produce; I bet you it's cheaper for them than it would be for you!

~ Always try something new! We've tried all kinds of "strange" and new things at the market, and loved the experience of trying each and every one. From goose eggs to bitter melon, make it a culinary adventure your kids can help you conquer.

We've gotten to know a lot of local growers and even made friends at the market. We've been surprised at how affordable it can be, too. We end up using what we get, rather than overbuying produce at the grocery store and having items go to waste. When you see a beautiful butternut squash come into season, you're thrilled to be able to try new recipes, rather than taking it all for granted. Give it a try and you'll be sure to keep at it.

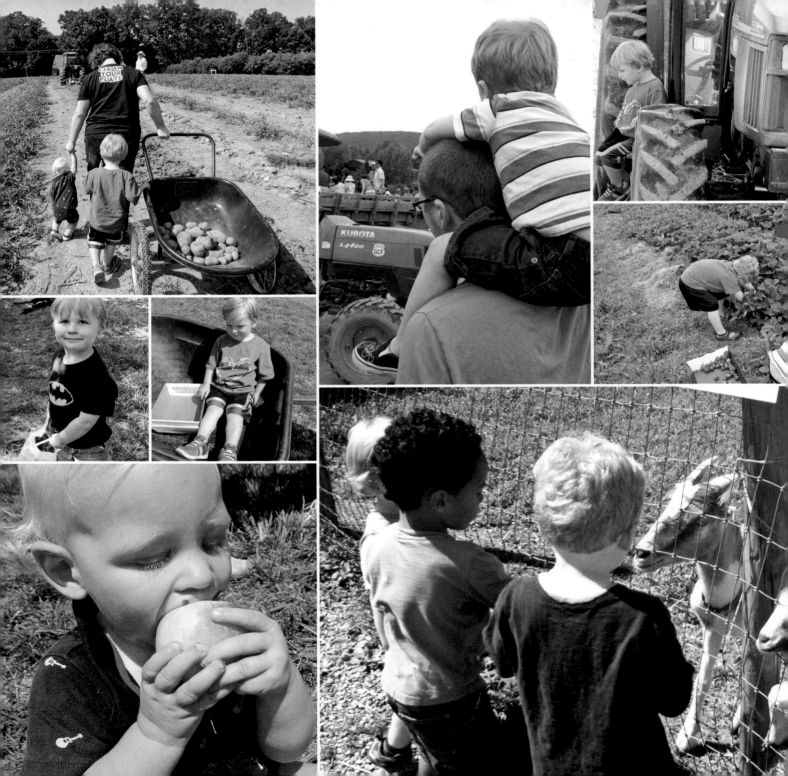

U-PICK FARMS

In our area, there are a few U-Pick farms that we visit every couple of weeks to find the fruits and vegetables that are in season. To encourage family attendance, most farms even have activities or seasonal festivals for kids to enjoy after they finish their picking. One of our farms is equipped with a giant jumping pillow and huge playgrounds; we pack a picnic and make it an all-day activity when the weather is nice. With a year-round membership, it's endless entertainment for the price of affordable, local, pesticide-free produce.

While at the farm picking, the children get to see what real food looks like in its natural state, and they come to appreciate the hard work farmers put in to get it to our table. Farming can be a lot of fun, too. You can dig in the dirt for potatoes and carrots or stain your hands picking blackberries. You can climb trees picking peaches or ride in a wagon as other people hand you their picked cherries and apples for the crates. It's an outdoor paradise for kids.

Whatever you pick, pick a lot! The produce doesn't get any fresher—and often, any cheaper. We buy as much as we have the energy to pick (bushels are cheapest in bulk) and then freeze or store long term. Apples and potatoes last months on their own, and most fruits freeze wonderfully. That's what we use in our smoothies and our Maple Macadamia Cherry Crumble (p. 197)!

273

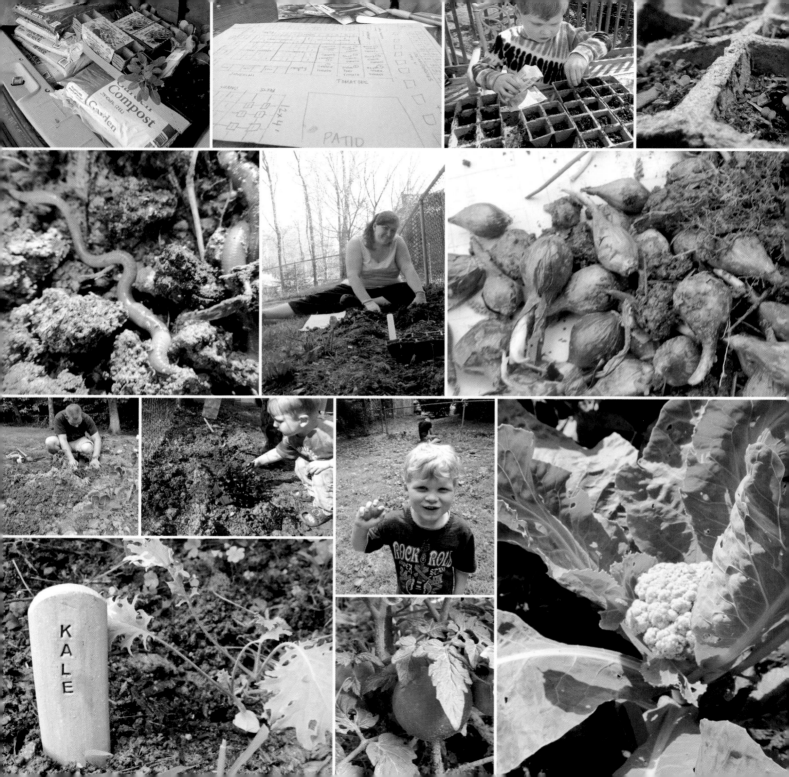

GARDENING

When we first moved into our house, we were excited to use our backyard to plant a garden and grow our own food. How awesome would it be to look outside our windows every day and see our plants growing higher and higher until we could pick them? The day we decided to start was very exciting for us. What were we going to grow? We needed a plan.

We made a list of everything we wanted to plant. Everyone chose a favorite: Cole needed zucchini and Finn wanted cantaloupe, while us parents wanted tomatoes, Brussels sprouts, and cauliflower. Matt tilled the area where we wanted to make our garden (measure beforehand and make sure your lines are straight!). We all helped spread soil and manure (it's horse poop and a little stinky, but plants and worms love it!) on top and then mixed the dirt again.

The best part was going to the gardening store and picking out our plants and seeds. While plants are more expensive than seeds, we're not the best gardeners. If a plant is really difficult to grow, you'll make your life a lot easier by getting it already potted. We like to plant the entire garden with biodegradable paper pots.

To get ready for planting, we made a map of our garden. Now, granted, we are organizers by nature, and maybe you don't need to do this. But it's easier to plant when you know where things go.

All seed packets explain how to plant the seeds, how far apart they should be, and what sunlight they need. So we mapped it all out with the space we had before we tilled the dirt. Then we planted our seeds, plants, and paper pots, marking them with garden markers. You have to label your plants somehow because they don't look like anything for a long time, and you need something to tell the weeds apart!

Then you just have to wait! And water. And wait some more. Pull weeds when they pop up, at least once at week, and check for ripe fruits and vegetables as often as you can. Nothing is cooler than seeing that first ripe tomato, picking it, and eating it for dinner that very night!

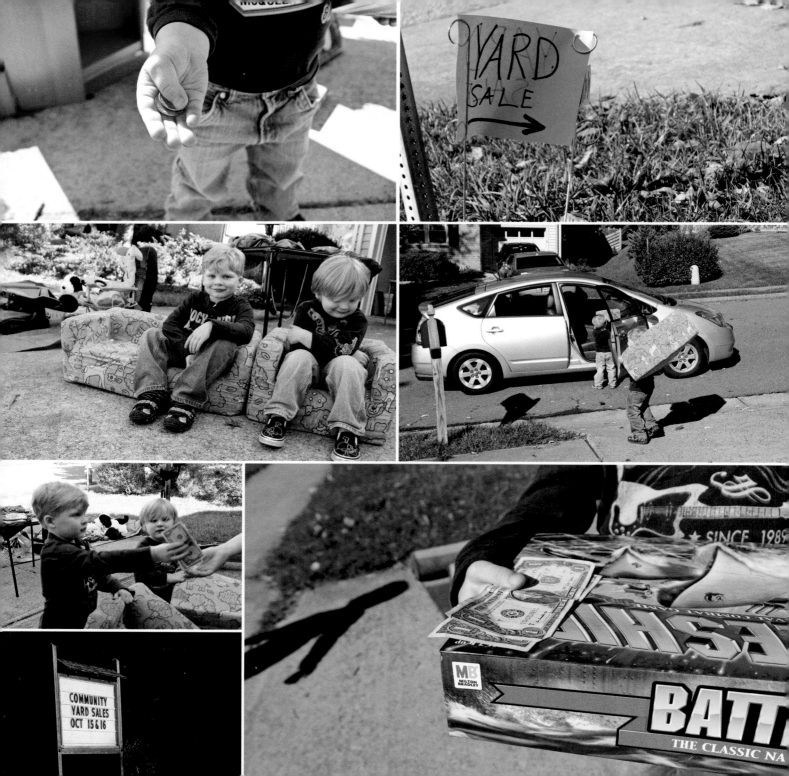

Yard Sales & Thrift Stores

Have you ever wanted to try something but found it too expensive? Maybe someone else down the street has that thing you want, never used it, and is looking to sell. Local yard sales and thrift stores bring people together so that nothing goes to waste and an affordable purchase can be made! We get lots of great stuff by simply shopping used; most of our kitchen appliances were purchased secondhand, and we're always happy to keep another item out of the landfill.

We've mentioned many somewhat unusual items in this book, like dehydrators, mandolins, meat grinders, and food processors. Most of the recipes we provided don't require these items, but they do make things much easier if you can find them. There are even more wonderful things we love but haven't mentioned in this book, such as a stick blender, deep fryer, and vegetable steamer. We have found all of these items from yard sales or thrift stores.

Thrift stores are easy to look up, but yard-saling (the verb of visiting yard sales) is a skill that takes a lifetime to master. Stacy's mother taught her young and she's been teaching the boys. The best thing to do is just drive around.

We like the nicest neighborhoods we can find, but the neighborhoods should be young enough for families to live there. Neighborhoods with older residents won't have items you commonly use, and trust me, older folks think their stuff is worth WAY more than it is and will tell you all about the item's history while your child attempts to crash their table of fine china. Find good neighborhoods and drive around and shop by signs. Have your kids help you look for the brightly colored posters and let them shop with a dollar for however many years old they are, if you are able. It's amazing what a three-year-old can get at yard sales!

The next best strategy for yard sales is to shop for specific items. Use Craigslist.com to search for "food processor" or "ice cream maker" and find the best listings. Decide where to try first based on the neighborhood and other sales around (Craigslist has a ton of listings every week). Then get there early (if it opens at 8 AM, be there at 7:50 AM) to score your deal. Use the Internet, look up local sales, make sure you have cash, and go! You'll have a lot of fun searching through everything, and we guarantee you will find things you didn't even know you needed!

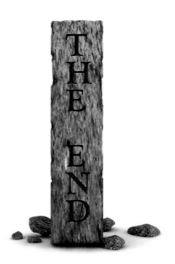

CONCLUSION

Recently, Cole came home from school excited by a "treat bag" he earned for good behavior. We were very proud of him. It wasn't that long ago, after all, that it would have been an "incident" report instead. Inside the bag were some stickers, a pencil, and three sugar candies. Cole took the pencil and the stickers and threw away the rest. When asked why, he replied: "I don't want candy. It makes me sick and it's unhealthy."

It took a year and a half to get him there, but here he is: healthy and strong, with a resolve to match. It was not always an easy journey, but it was one we all took together and came out on the other side the better for it.

We hope that you are using this book and changing your family for the better. The benefits you will see from eating a healthy diet are tremendous and will last a lifetime. Cooking, learning, and eating together has brought us closer as a family, and we know it will do the same for you.

And we hope that you get great joy from acting like a dinosaur with your kids!

278

RESOURCES

For Ingredients:

Grassfed Meats
US Wellness Meats
http://www.uswellnessmeats.com

Coconut Products
Tropical Traditions
http://tropicaltraditions.com

Almond Flour
Honeyville Food Products
http://www.honeyvillegrain.com

Lunchmeat
Applegate Farms
http://www.applegatefarms.com

U Pick Farms
http://www.upick.org

Grass Fed Farms
http://www.eatwild.com

For Lunchboxes:

Bento Boxes
http://www.laptoplunches.com

Goodbyns
http://www.goodbyn.com

Steel Containers
http://www.steeltainer.com

On Dietary Advice:

Robb Wolf
Http://www.robbwolf.com

Mark's Daily Apple
http://www.marksdailyapple.com

Balanced Bites
http://www.balancedbites.com

Cave Girl Eats
http://www.cavegirleats.com

For More Recipes:

The Food Lovers' Primal Palate
www.primal-palate.com

Nom Nom Paleo
http://www.nomnompaleo.com

Elana's Pantry
http://www.Elanaspantry.com

To Visit Us:

To visit us:
http://www.paleoparents.com
http://www.facebook.com/paleoparents
http://www.twitter.com/paleoparents

INGREDIENT INDEX

MAIN DISHES ALLERGEN GUIDE
*ALL RECIPES FREE OF DAIRY, WHEAT, PEANUTS, AND SOY

		fish	shellfish	tree nuts	eggs
50/50 Bacon Burgers	p. 51	NO	NO	NO	NO
Shakey Pork Barbecue	p. 53	NO	NO	NO	NO
Pulled Pork	p. 55	NO	NO	NO	NO
Pork Roast with Squishy Squashy Apples	p. 57	NO	NO	NO	NO
Fried Cauli Rice with Shrimp	p. 59	YES	YES	NO	YES
Fish in a Boat and Cole's Salmon Salad	p. 61	YES	NO	NO	YES
Lemon Dill Salmon	p. 63	YES	NO	NO	NO
Curried Mussels, Not Muscles	p. 65	NO	YES	NO	NO
Mini Egg Pizzas	p. 67	NO	NO	NO	YES
Goose Egg Scramble	p. 69	NO	NO	NO	YES
Eggs in a Nest	p. 71	NO	NO	NO	YES
Sweet Quiche	p. 73	NO	NO	NO	YES
Kale, Bacon, & Black Olive Egg Pie	p. 75	NO	NO	NO	YES
Egg Salad	p. 77	NO	NO	NO	YES
Maple Chicken Salad	p. 79	NO	NO	NO	YES
Fool's Gold (Chicken Nuggets)	p. 81	NO	NO	YES	NO
Hissin' Chicken	p. 83	NO	NO	NO	NO
Steak & Strawberry Salad	p. 85	NO	NO	NO	NO
Meatball Salad	p. 87	NO	NO	NO	YES
Pineapple Curry	p. 89	YES	NO	NO	NO
Beef & Broccoli	p. 91	NO	NO	NO	NO
Spaghetti with Meatballs	p. 93	NO	NO	NO	NO
Shepherd's Pie	p. 95	NO	NO	NO	NO
Halupki Casserole	p. 97	NO	NO	NO	NO
Rat on a Stick	p. 99	NO	NO	NO	YES
Roast Beast	p. 101	NO	NO	NO	NO

Eat Like a Dinosaur

SIDE DISHES ALLERGEN GUIDE
*ALL RECIPES FREE OF DAIRY, WHEAT, PEANUTS, AND SOY

		fish	shellfish	tree nuts	eggs
Deviled Bacony Eggs	p. 105	NO	NO	NO	YES
Ratatouille	p. 107	NO	NO	NO	NO
Carrot Rounds	p. 109	NO	NO	NO	NO
Bunny's Soup	p. 111	NO	NO	NO	NO
Zucchini Latkes	p. 113	NO	NO	NO	YES
Little Cabbage (Brussels Sprouts)	p. 115	NO	NO	NO	NO
Chou Vert (Big Cabbage)	p. 117	NO	NO	NO	NO
Nature's Spears (Asparagus)	p. 119	NO	NO	NO	NO
Greens & Bacon	p. 121	NO	NO	NO	NO
Roasted Sweet Potatoes	p. 123	NO	NO	NO	NO
Maple Butternut Squash Purée	p. 125	NO	NO	NO	NO
Sweet Potato Fries	p. 127	NO	NO	NO	NO
Apple Bacon Slaw	p. 129	NO	NO	NO	NO
Applesauce	p. 131	NO	NO	NO	NO
Bone Stock	p. 133	NO	NO	NO	NO

DIPS AND SAUCES ALLERGEN GUIDE
*ALL RECIPES FREE OF DAIRY, WHEAT, PEANUTS, AND SOY

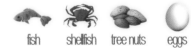

		fish	shellfish	tree nuts	eggs
Mayonnaise	p. 137	NO	NO	NO	YES
Mock-a-Mole	p. 139	NO	NO	NO	NO
Black Olive Tapenade	p. 141	NO	NO	YES	NO
Ten Tomato Ketchup	p. 143	NO	NO	NO	NO
Texas Barbecue Sauce	p. 145	NO	NO	NO	NO
Raspberry Dressing	p. 147	NO	NO	NO	NO
Southwestern Pineapple Sauce	p. 149	NO	NO	NO	NO
Savory Coconut Cream Sauce	p. 151	NO	NO	NO	NO
Thai Curry Coconut Dip	p. 153	NO	NO	NO	NO

Eat Like a Dinosaur

SNACKS ALLERGEN GUIDE
*ALL RECIPES FREE OF DAIRY, WHEAT, PEANUTS, AND SOY

		fish	shellfish	tree nuts	eggs
Teriyaki Beef Jerky	p. 157	NO	NO	NO	NO
Tacos to Go (Chicken Jerky)	p. 159	NO	NO	NO	NO
Honey Barbecue Ground Jerky	p. 161	NO	NO	NO	NO
Kale Chips	p. 163	NO	NO	NO	NO
Apple Rings	p. 165	NO	NO	NO	NO
Cinnamon Apple Tidbits	p. 167	NO	NO	NO	NO
Rolled Fruit Leathers	p. 169	NO	NO	NO	NO
Anytime Cookies	p. 171	NO	NO	YES	NO
Graham Cookies	p. 173	NO	NO	YES	YES
Grain-Free Granola	p. 175	NO	NO	YES	NO
Candied Nuts	p. 177	NO	NO	YES	NO
Cherry Chocolate Balls	p. 179	NO	NO	YES	NO
Pumpkin Cider "Latte"	p. 181	NO	NO	NO	NO
Elvis's Nut Butter and Nana Smoothie	p. 183	NO	NO	YES	NO
Hawaiian Vacation Smoothie	p. 185	NO	NO	YES	NO
Pineapple, Mint, and Clementine Water	p. 187	NO	NO	NO	NO

SPECIAL TREATS ALLERGEN GUIDE
*ALL RECIPES FREE OF DAIRY, WHEAT, PEANUTS, AND SOY

		fish	shellfish	tree nuts	eggs
Chocolate Chip Cookies	p. 191	NO	NO	YES	YES
Chocolate Milkshake	p. 193	NO	NO	NO	NO
Mini Nut Butter Cups	p. 195	NO	NO	NO	YES
Cherry Macadamia Crumble	p. 197	NO	NO	YES	YES
Banana Chocolate Chip Bread	p. 199	NO	NO	NO	YES
Banana Bubble Pudding	p. 201	NO	NO	NO	NO
Whipped Coconut Cream	p. 203	NO	NO	NO	NO
Coconut Cream Pie	p. 205	NO	NO	YES	YES
Pie Crust	p. 207	NO	NO	YES	NO
Samoa Cake Balls	p. 209	NO	NO	YES	YES
German Chocolate Cake Balls	p. 211	NO	NO	YES	YES
Lava Fudge Cupcakes	p. 213	NO	NO	YES	YES
Chocolate Fudge Frosting	p. 215	NO	NO	NO	NO
Apple Pie Cupcakes	p. 217	NO	NO	YES	YES
Caramel Icing	p. 219	NO	NO	NO	NO
Gigi's Carrot Cupcakes	p. 221	NO	NO	YES	YES
ZuCakes	p. 223	NO	NO	YES	YES
Red Brownie Cupcakes	p. 225	NO	NO	YES	YES
Creamy Not Cheese Frosting	p. 227	NO	NO	YES	NO
Pumpkin Pucks	p. 229	NO	NO	YES	YES
Frozen Waffles	p. 231	NO	NO	NO	YES
Cinnamon Apple Creamed Hot Cereal	p. 233	NO	NO	YES	NO
Watermelon Ice Pops	p. 235	NO	NO	NO	NO
Honey Nut Ice Cream	p. 237	NO	NO	YES	NO
Mint Chocolate Chip Ice Cream	p. 239	NO	NO	NO	NO
Chocolate Nut Butter Ripple Ice Cream	p. 241	NO	NO	NO	NO
Caramel Sauce	p. 243	NO	NO	NO	NO
Fudge Sauce	p. 245	NO	NO	NO	NO

Eat Like a Dinosaur